PEDIATRICS, CHILD AND ADOLESCENT HEALTH

MULTIPLE SCLEROSIS IN CHILDREN AND ADOLESCENTS

Pediatrics, Child and Adolescent Health

Joav Merrick - Series Editor

National Institute of Child Health
and Human Development,
Ministry of Social Affairs, Jerusalem

Multiple Sclerosis in Children and Adolescents
Hatim Omar, MD and Joshua Chalkley
2017. ISBN: 978-1-53612-979-3 (Hardcover)
2017. ISBN: 978-1-53612-980-9 (e-book)

Positive Youth Development: Long Term Effects in a Chinese Program
Daniel TL Shek, Cecilia MS Ma, Janet TY Leung and Joav Merrick (Editors)
2017. ISBN: 978-1-53612-539-9 (Hardcover)
2017. ISBN: 978-1-53612-540-5 (e-book)

Bicycles: Helmet Use of Adolescents at Independent Schools
Ronald Chow, Michael Borean, Drew Hollenberg, Jaclyn Viehweger, Tharani Anpalagan and Anna Rzepka (Editors)
2017. ISBN: 978-1-53612-458-3 (Softcover)
2017. ISBN: 978-1-53612-459-0 (e-book)

Adolescence: Bicycle and Helmet Use of Adolescents and Young Adults
Ronald Chow and Joav Merrick (Editors)
2017. ISBN: 978-1-53612-039-4 (Hardcover)
2017. ISBN: 978-1-53612-060-8 (e-book)

Suicide: A Global View on Suicidal Ideation among Adolescents
Mazyanga L. Mazaba, Seter Siziya and Joav Merrick (Editors)
2017. ISBN: 978-1-53611-788-2 (Hardcover)
2017. ISBN: 978-1-53611-799-8 (e-book)

Children and Youth: Post-Traumatic Stress Disorder and Motor Vehicle Crashes
Donald E. Greydanus, Roger W. Apple, Kathryn White, and Joav Merrick (Editors
2017. ISBN: 978-1-53611-102-6 (Hardcover)
2017. ISBN: 978-1-53611-255-9 (e-book)

Child and Adolescent Health Yearbook 2016
Joav Merrick (Editor)
2017. ISBN: 978-1-53610-948-1 (Hardcover)
2017. ISBN: 978-1-53610-957-3 (e-book)

Child Health and Human Development Yearbook 2016
Joav Merrick (Editor)
2017. ISBN: 978-1-53610-946-7 (Hardcover)
2017. ISBN: 978-1-53610-958-0 (e-book)

Chronic Disease and Disability: The Pediatric Kidney
Donald E Greydanus, Vimal Master Sankar Raj, and Joav Merrick (Editors)
2016. ISBN: 978-1-63483-793-4 (Hardcover)
2015. ISBN: 978-1-63483-809-2 (e-book)

Child and Adolescent Health Yearbook 2015
Joav Merrick (Editor)
2016. ISBN: 978-1-63484-512-0 (Hardcover)
2016. ISBN: 978-1-63484-543-4 (e-book)

Child Health and Human Development Yearbook 2015
Joav Merrick (Editor)
2016. ISBN: 978-1-63484-513-7 (Hardcover)
2016. ISBN: 978-1-63484-544-1 (e-book)

Pain Management Yearbook 2015
Joav Merrick (Editor)
2016. ISBN: 978-1-63484-515-1 (Hardcover)
2016. ISBN: 978-1-63484-545-8 (e-book)

Children and Childhood: Some International Aspects
Joav Merrick (Editor)
2016. ISBN: 978-1-63484-587-8 (Hardcover)
2016. ISBN: 978-1-63484-594-6 (e-book)

Children and Adolescents: Future Challenges
Daniel TL Shek, Tak Yan Lee, and Joav Merrick (Editors)
2016. ISBN: 978-1-63484-616-5 (Hardcover)
2016. ISBN: 978-1-63484-627-1 (e-book)

Adolescence: Positive Youth Development Programs in Chinese Communities
Daniel TL Shek, Florence KY Wu, Janet TY Leung, and Joav Merrick (Editors)
2016. ISBN: 978-1-63484-044-6 (Hardcover)
2016. ISBN: 978-1-63484-677-6 (e-book)

Sexuality: Some International Aspects
Joav Merrick and Donald E Greydanus (Editors)
2016. ISBN: 978-1-63484-707-0 (Hardcover)
2016. ISBN: 978-1-63484-719-3 (e-book)

Growing Up in the Middle East: The Daily Lives and Well-Being of Israeli and Palestinian Youth
Yossi Harel-Fisch, Ziad Abdeen and Miriam Navot
2016. ISBN: 978-1-63484-746-9 (Hardcover)
2016. ISBN: 978-1-63484-765-0 (e-book)

Chronic Disease and Disability: The Pediatric Heart
Donald E Greydanus, Devika Malhotra and Joav Merrick (Editors)
2016. ISBN: 978-1-63484-828-2 (Hardcover)
2016. ISBN: 978-1-63484-842-8 (e-book)

Diabetes Mellitus: Childhood and Adolescence
Manmohan K Kamboj, Donald E Greydanus and Joav Merrick (Editors)
2016. ISBN: 978-1-53610-095-2 (Hardcover)
2016. ISBN: 978-1-53610-104-1 (e-book)

Chronic Disease and Disability: Abuse and Neglect in Childhood and Adolescence
Donald E Greydanus, Vincent J Palusci and Joav Merrick (Editors)
2016. ISBN: 978-1-53610-129-4 (Hardcover)
2016. ISBN: 978-1-53610-142-3 (e-book)

Clinical Aspects of Psychopharmacology in Childhood and Adolescence, Second Edition
Donald E Greydanus, Joseph L Calles, Jr, Dilip R Patel, Ahsan Nazeer and Joav Merrick (Editors)
2016. ISBN: 978-1-53610-241-3 (Hardcover)
2016. ISBN: 978-1-53610-253-6 (e-book)

Chronic Disease and Disability: The Pediatric Pancreas
Donald E Greydanus, Manmohan K Kamboj and Joav Merrick (Editors)
2016. ISBN: 978-1-53610-055-6 (Hardcover)
2016. ISBN: 978-1-53610-065-5 (e-book)

A Pediatric Resident Pocket Guide: Making the Most of Morning Reports
Arthur N Feinberg
2015. ISBN: 978-1-63482-141-4 (Softcover)
2015. ISBN: 978-1-63482-186-5 (e-book)

Tropical Pediatrics: A Public Health Concern of International Proportions Second Edition
Richard R Roach, Donald E Greydanus, Dilip R Patel and Joav Merrick (Editors)
2015. ISBN: 978-1-63463-381-9 (Hardcover)
2015. ISBN: 978-1-63463-404-5 (e-book)

Child and Adolescent Health Issues (A Tribute to the Pediatrician Donald E Greydanus)
Joav Merrick (Editor)
2015. ISBN: 978-1-63463-574-5 (Hardcover)
2015. ISBN: 978-1-63463-576-9 (e-book)

Child and Adolescent Health Yearbook 2014
Joav Merrick (Editor)
2015. ISBN: 978-1-63482-162-9 (Hardcover)
2015. ISBN: 978-1-63482-206-0 (e-book)

Child Health and Human Development Yearbook 2014
Joav Merrick (Editor)
2015. ISBN: 978-1-63482-163-6 (Hardcover)
2015. ISBN: 978-1-63482-207-7 (e-book)

Behavioral Pediatrics, 4th Edition
Donald E Greydanus, Dilip R Patel, Helen D Pratt, Joseph L Calles Jr, Ahsan Nazeer and Joav Merrick (Editors)
2015. ISBN: 978-1-63483-027-0 (Hardcover)
2015. ISBN: 978-1-63483-052-2 (e-book)

Disability, Chronic Disease and Human Development
Joav Merrick
2015. ISBN: 978-1-63483-029-4 (Hardcover)
2015. ISBN: 978-1-63483-057-7 (e-book)

Caribbean Adolescents: Some Public Health Concerns
Cecilia Hegamin-Younge and Joav Merrick (Editors)
2015. ISBN: 978-1-63483-341-7 (Hardcover)
2015. ISBN: 978-1-63483-343-1 (e-book)

Adolescence and Health: Some International Perspectives
Joav Merrick (Editor)
2015. ISBN: 978-1-63483-791-0 (Hardcover)
2015. ISBN: 978-1-63483-808-5 (e-book)

Youth Suicide Prevention: Everybody's Business
Hatim A Omar (Editor)
2015. ISBN: 978-1-63483-786-6 (Softcover)
2015. ISBN: 978-1-63483-820-7 (e-book)

Human Developmental Research: Experience from Research in Hong Kong
Daniel TL Shek, Cecilia Ma, Yu Lu and Joav Merrick (Editors)
2014. ISBN: 978-1-62808-166-4 (Hardcover)
2013. ISBN: 978-1-62808-167-1 (e-book)

School, Adolescence and Health Issues
Joav Merrick, Ariel Tenenbaum and Hatim A Omar (Editors)
2014. ISBN: 978-1-62948-702-1 (Hardcover)
2014. ISBN: 978-1-62948-707-6 (e-book)

Adolescence and Sexuality: International Perspectives
Joav Merrick, Ariel Tenenbaum and Hatim A Omar (Editors)
2014. ISBN: 978-1-62948-711-3 (Hardcover)
2014. ISBN: 978-1-62948-724-3 (e-book)

Child and Adolescent Health Yearbook 2013
Joav Merrick (Editor)
2014. ISBN: 978-1-63117-658-6 (Hardcover)
2014. ISBN: 978-1-63117-668-5 (e-book)

Adoption: The Search for a New Parenthood
Gary Diamond and Eva Arbel (Israel)
2014. ISBN: 978-1-63117-710-1 (Hardcover)
2014. ISBN: 978-1-63117-713-2 (e-book)

Adolescence: Places and Spaces
Myra F Taylor, Julie Ann Pooley and Joav Merrick (Editors)
2014. ISBN: 978-1-63117-847-4 (Hardcover)
2014. ISBN: 978-1-63117-850-4 (e-book)

Pain Management Yearbook 2013
Joav Merrick (Editor)
2014. ISBN: 978-1-63117-944-0 (Hardcover)
2014. ISBN: 978-1-63117-959-4 (e-book)

Child Health and Human Development Yearbook 2013
Joav Merrick (Editor)
2014. ISBN: 978-1-63117-939-6 (Hardcover)
2013. ISBN: 978-1-63117-958-7 (e-book)

Born into this World: Health Issues
Donald E Greydanus, Arthur N Feinberg, and Joav Merrick (Editors)
2014. ISBN: 978-1-63321-667-9 (Hardcover)
2014. ISBN: 978-1-63321-669-3 (e-book)

Caring for the Newborn: A Comprehensive Guide for the Clinician
Donald E Greydanus, Arthur N Feinberg and Joav Merrick (Editors)
2014. ISBN: 978-1-63321-760-7 (Hardcover)
2014. ISBN: 978-1-63321-781-2 (e-book)

Environment and Hope: Improving Health, Reducing AIDS and Promoting Food Security in the World
Leslie Rubin and Joav Merrick (Editors)
2014. ISBN: 978-1-63321-772-0 (Hardcover)
2014. ISBN: 978-1-63321-782-9 (e-book)

Pediatric and Adolescent Dermatology: Some Current Issues
Donald E Greydanus, Arthur N Feinberg and Joav Merrick (Editors)
2014. ISBN: 978-1-63321-853-6 (Hardcover)
2014. ISBN: 978-1-63321-863-5 (e-book)

Adolescence and Behavior Issues in a Chinese Context
Daniel TL Shek, Rachel CF Sun, and Joav Merrick (Editors)
2013. ISBN: 978-1-62618-614-9 (Hardcover)
2013. ISBN: 978-1-62618-692-7 (e-book)

Advances in Preterm Infant Research
Jing Sun, Nicholas Buys and Joav Merrick
2013. ISBN: 978-1-62618-696-5 (Hardcover)
2013. ISBN: 978-1-62618-775-7 (e-book)

Child Health and Human Development: Social, Economic and Environmental Factors
Leslie Rubin and Joav Merrick (Editors)
2013. ISBN: 978-1-62948-166-1 (Hardcover)
2013. ISBN: 978-1-62948-169-2 (e-book)

Children, Violence and Bullying: International Perspectives
Joav Merrick, Isack Kandel and Hatim A Omar (Editors)
2013. ISBN: 978-1-62948-342-9 (Hardcover)
2013. ISBN: 978-1-62948-345-0 (e-book)

Chinese Adolescent Development: Economic Disadvantages, Parents and Intrapersonal Development
Daniel TL Shek, Rachel CF Sun and Joav Merrick (Editors)
2013. ISBN: 978-1-62618-622-4 (Hardcover)
2013. ISBN: 978-1-62618-694-1 (e-book)

Chronic Disease and Disability in Childhood
Joav Merrick
2013. ISBN: 978-1-62808-865-6 (Hardcover)
2013. ISBN: 978-1-62808-868-7 (e-book)

Environmental Health Disparities in Children: Asthma, Obesity and Food
Leslie Rubin and Joav Merrick (Editors)
2013. ISBN: 978-1-62948-122-7 (Hardcover)
2013. ISBN: 978-1-62948-135-7 (e-book)

Environmental Health: Home, School and Community
Leslie Rubin and Joav Merrick (Editors)
2013. ISBN: 978-1-62948-155-5 (Hardcover)
2013. ISBN: 978-1-62948-158-6 (e-book)

Guidelines for the Healthy Integration of the Ill Child in the Educational System: Experience from Israel
Yosefa Isenberg
2013. ISBN: 978-1-62808-350-7 (Hardcover)
2013. ISBN: 978-1-62808-353-8 (e-book)

Internet Addiction: A Public Health Concern in Adolescence
Artemis Tsitsika, Mari Janikian, Donald E Greydanus, Hatim A Omar and Joav Merrick (Editors)
2013. ISBN: 978-1-62618-925-6 (Hardcover)
2013. ISBN: 978-1-62618-959-1 (e-book)

Playing with Fire: Children, Adolescents and Firesetting
Hatim A. Omar, Carrie Howell Bowling and Joav Merrick (Editors)
2013. ISBN: 978-1-62948-471-6 (Softcover)
2013. ISBN: 978-1-62948-474-7 (e-book)

Promotion of Holistic Development of Young People in Hong Kong
Daniel TL Shek, Tak Yan Lee and Joav Merrick (Editors)
2013. ISBN: 978-1-62808-019-3 (Hardcover)
2013. ISBN: 978-1-62808-040-7 (e-book)

University and College Students: Health and Development Issues for the Leaders of Tomorrow
Daniel TL Shek, Rachel CF and Joav Merrick (Editors)
2013. ISBN: 978-1-62618-586-9 (Hardcover)
2013. ISBN: 978-1-62618-612-5 (e-book)

Break the Cycle of Environmental Health Disparities: Maternal and Child Health Aspects
Leslie Rubin and Joav Merrick (Editors)
2013. ISBN: 978-1-62948-107-4 (Hardcover)
2013. ISBN: 978-1-62948-133-3 (e-book)

Child and Adolescent Health Yearbook 2012
Joav Merrick (Editor)
2012. ISBN: 978-1-61942-788-4 (Hardcover)
2012. ISBN: 978-1-61942-789-1 (e-book)

Child Health and Human Development Yearbook 2011
Joav Merrick (Editor)
2012. ISBN: 978-1-61942-969-7 (Hardcover)
2012. ISBN: 978-1-61942-970-3 (e-book)

Child and Adolescent Health Yearbook 2011
Joav Merrick (Editor)
2012. ISBN: 978-1-61942-782-2 (Hardcover)
2012. ISBN: 978-1-61942-783-9 (e-book)

Tropical Pediatrics: A Public Health Concern of International Proportions
Richard R Roach, Donald E Greydanus, Dilip R Patel, Douglas N Homnick and Joav Merrick (Editors)
2012. ISBN: 978-1-61942-831-7 (Hardcover)
2012. ISBN: 978-1-61942-840-9 (e-book)

Child Health and Human Development Yearbook 2012
Joav Merrick (Editor)
2012. ISBN: 978-1-61942-978-9 (Hardcover)
2012. ISBN: 978-1-61942-979-6 (e-book)

Developmental Issues in Chinese Adolescents
Daniel TL Shek, Rachel CF Sun and Joav Merrick (Editors)
2012. ISBN: 978-1-62081-262-4 (Hardcover)
2012. ISBN: 978-1-62081-270-9 (e-book)

Positive Youth Development: Theory, Research and Application
Daniel TL Shek, Rachel CF Sun and Joav Merrick (Editors)
2012. ISBN: 978-1-62081-305-8 (Hardcover)
2012. ISBN: 978-1-62081-347-8 (e-book)

Positive Youth Development: A New School Curriculum to Tackle Adolescent Developmental Issues
Hing Keung Ma, Daniel TL Shek and Joav Merrick (Editors)
2012. ISBN: 978-1-62081-384-3 (Hardcover)
2012. ISBN: 978-1-62081-385-0 (e-book)

Understanding Autism Spectrum Disorder: Current Research Aspects
Ditza A Zachor and Joav Merrick (Editors)
2012. ISBN: 978-1-62081-353-9 (Hardcover)
2012. ISBN: 978-1-62081-390-4 (e-book)

Transition from Pediatric to Adult Medical Care
David Wood, John G Reiss, Maria E Ferris, Linda R Edwards and Joav Merrick (Editors)
2012. ISBN: 978-1-62081-409-3 (Hardcover)
2012. ISBN: 978-1-62081-412-3 (e-book)

PEDIATRICS, CHILD AND ADOLESCENT HEALTH

MULTIPLE SCLEROSIS IN CHILDREN AND ADOLESCENTS

HATIM OMAR
AND
JOSHUA CHALKLEY
EDITORS

nova biomedical
New York

Library of Congress Cataloging-in-Publication Data

ISBN: 978-1-53612-979-3

Published by Nova Science Publishers, Inc. † New York

DEDICATION

This book is dedicated to my amazing son, Kareem, who at 19 years of age has accomplished more than many people will in a life time. He has been a delight to raise and a great young man to hang out with. A Governor's Scholar, a Presidential Scholar, a pilot, a NASA affiliated researcher and a straight A student, while still being caring, loving and helpful. When all his good deeds were rewarded with a life-changing diagnosis of multiple sclerosis, he took it in stride and showed courage and determination in the face of adversity. I love you son and I am proud of you.

This is also dedicated to my wife Youlia who is an outstanding mother that was always there to support Kareem and encourage him and make his life easier.

Hatim Omar, MD
Editor

CONTENTS

FOREWORD

*Joshua Chalkley**, *DO MS*
Department of Neurology, Neuroimmunology/MS Division,
University of Kentucky, Lexington, KY, US

We are currently undergoing a revolution in the treatment of multiple sclerosis. The first effective treatments for MS were introduced in the early 1990s, and over the last decade new treatment options continue to abound. In a disease which used to lead to serious disability in most patients after a decade we now consider no evidence of disease activity the gold standard of treatment (although still not reaching this goal as much as we would like). Despite these advances the treatment of pediatric multiple sclerosis has lagged behind the adult literature. Pediatric MS was thought to be vanishingly rare. Increasingly, pediatric multiple sclerosis is being recognized, we have started to study pediatric MS in a systematic way. The first clinical trials for pediatric MS are underway, and hopefully within the next decade we will have good clinical trial data for the treatment of pediatric MS.

---

* Correspondence: Joshua Chalkley DO, MS. Assistant Professor of Neurology, Neuroimmunology/MS Division. University of Kentucky. 740 South Limestone, Lexington, KY. E-mail: Josh.Chalkley@uky.edu.

I would like to thank all the physicians who contributed to this book, I am in their debt for their time and expertise. It was a pleasure working with such a talented group of pediatricians, neurologists, and pediatric neurologists who dedicated their time in the writing of this book. It is truly a pleasure to have access to so many stellar colleagues whose knowledge, clinical acumen, technical skill, and compassion continue to inspire me to be a better doctor. I would be amiss if I did thank my mentors who spent so much time teaching me the field. Dr. Berger, Dr. Weiner, Dr. Stankiewicz, Dr. Severson, Dr. Baskshi, Dr. Kimbrough Dr. Chitnis, just to name a few your guidance and wisdom is much appreciated. I would also like to thank the patients who are often dealing with difficult circumstances. Our ultimate hope is the propagation of knowledge leads to the alleviation of suffering, why else be a doctor. We are forever in your debt.

INTRODUCTION

Hatim Omar*, MD

Division of Adolescent Medicine and Young Parent Programs, Kentucky Clinic, Department of Pediatrics, Kentucky Children's Hospital, University of Kentucky College of Medicine, Lexington, KY, US

Multiple sclerosis (MS) is often an afterthought when primary care providers and even some neurologists when doing initial evaluation of a young person with what seems to be a neuromuscular disease. It is usually low on the differential diagnosis list which unfortunately delays proper diagnosis and early treatment. As a provider caring for children and adolescents, I am sure I was just as oblivious to the incidence of MS in this age group. A few years ago, my son, 18 years of age at the time, called me and indicated that he lost sensation in his legs but no muscle weakness. He went to student health then to the emergency department in the city where he lived on college campus, and was told in both places not to worry about it, probably a viral infection. I knew that my son never really complained and if he was concerned then it must be serious. He then went to see a

* Correspondence: Hatim Omar, MD. Department of Pediatrics, Division of Adolescent Medicine. 740 S. Limestone, Lexington, KY 40536. E-mail: haomar2@uky.edu.

neurologist, who promptly diagnosed him with Guillain-Barré syndrome, because it was 2 days after receiving flu vaccine (even though the vaccine was live flu that has not been associated with this syndrome). I never felt comfortable with the diagnosis as a dad or a physician and thus asked for evaluation at a different institution where the diagnosis of MS was given.

Many of us in health care also, are not fully aware of the financial, psychosocial and insurance problems facing these patients and their families which can and do impact the outcome.

This book is a humble contribution targeted at primary care providers as a brief handy reference to help prevent late diagnosis and treatment. It is not intended for specialists who work with multiple sclerosis regularly

PREFACE

Multiple Sclerosis is one of the most common neurological disorders leading to disability. Many cases of Multiple Sclerosis are diagnosed late especially in young patients because providers are not considering it early in their assessment and differential diagnosis. This book will provide an additional resource to health care providers working with children and adolescents to facilitate increased awareness and earlier diagnosis and treatment.

Chapter 1 - Multiple sclerosis initially thought to be disease of adults is invariably present in younger age groups as well. Most of the studies looking at pathophysiology of multiple sclerosis are based on adult patient population. Traditionally T cells were thought to be main immunological factor playing vital role in pathophysiology but recent studies suggest more complex picture involving roles of B cell, antibodies and innate immunity. Since MS is chronic inflammatory neurodegenerative disease and it's widely accepted that immune system of pediatric age group is different than adult counterparts hence a different pathophysiological model may be present. Many genetic and environmental factors play as etiological factors in MS. More research is needed to understand pathophysiology of multiple sclerosis in pediatric age group and looking into genetic and environmental etiological factors may broaden the horizon in understanding multiple sclerosis and may help in future research and treatment.

Chapter 2 - Differentiating Multiple Sclerosis from other demyelinating disorders can be extremely challenging, but is important as these disorders can have high neurologic morbidity. With advancing treatment options, early diagnosis is more important than ever.

Chapter 3 - Pediatric multiple sclerosis is very uncommon and clinical presentations, particularly in pre-adolescent patients, can vary dramatically as compared to post adolescent or adult manifestations of disease. The purpose of this chapter is to compare and contrast these differences by the authors' clinical experience/patient vignettes and review the literature.

Chapter 4 - The treatment of multiple sclerosis has undergone a major revolution over the last decade. In many patients, clinicians are able to keep the disease under control, however the literature in pediatric disease has lagged behind its adult counterparts. The purpose of this paper is to review the literature on the treatment of pediatric multiple sclerosis and to discuss developing treatment approaches in dealing with the pediatric population.

Chapter 5 - Pediatric onset multiple sclerosis (POMS) causes impairment in multiple domains, including physical, cognitive, and social. Physical disability is initially subtle and develops later in the course of the disease. Cognitive impairment is frequent and should be monitored closely. Fatigue and mood disorders occur as frequently in children as in adults with multiple sclerosis. All of these can have long-term effects on a child's quality of life, academic, and social functioning. When comparing patients with POMS to those with adult-onset disease of the same chronological age, those with POMS have poorer outcomes.

Chapter 6 - Symptom management is an integral part of the care of patients with multiple sclerosis. Complementary and alternative treatments have been mostly used for the management of symptoms in this patient population. The purpose of this paper is to review the literature on the various treatment modalities and available data supporting their use.

Chapter 7 - Multiple sclerosis (MS) is not a common diagnosis found in the pediatric population. Only 5% of those diagnosed with MS are in the pediatric age category. Due to the stage of development and impaired coping skills, adolescents are at high risk of negative outcomes when given an MS diagnosis. It is imperative for these teens to have strong positive support from parents, peers, school officials, and medical providers to ensure a good outcome. This chapter explores potential negative psychosocial outcomes in adolescents with MS and the interventions shown to be effective in prevention.

Chapter 8 - Pediatric multiple sclerosis affects not only the individual but also significantly affects family and friends. Roles and relationships may change. Parents or guardians must take on the role of caregiver for a child or adolescent with multiple sclerosis in addition to their parenting and child-rearing duties. A hallmark of multiple sclerosis is relapsing and remitting symptoms. However, some symptoms do not remit and become chronic. An individual may become affected in many ways including sensation, hearing, vision, speech, and movement. As a result, physical, social, and economic effects are an inevitable part of the disease. Good support is critical for the individual with multiple sclerosis, their family and caretakers, and their friends.

Chapter 9 - Pediatric multiple sclerosis (MS) is a chronic and debilitating disease associated with frequent hospitalizations and high health care costs. Although the diagnosis of pediatric MS is a relatively new and rare, steps must be taken in the future to reduce the substantial costs to the United States health care system and families suffering from effects of this disease. Direct and indirect costs related to pediatric MS include hospitalizations, diagnostic testing, drug therapy, missed school, and parental leave from work. Accurate and timely diagnosis, reduction in the cost of treatment, adequate health care coverage, and an understanding of the financial burden of MS are important steps in improvement of its monetary impact. A great deal of attention and research is required to address and decrease the financial burden of pediatric MS.

Chapter 10 - Multiple sclerosis is a chronic, debilitating autoimmune condition with unknown etiology. It can have significant impact on quality of life and overall sense of wellbeing. It can be associated with poor sleep, fatigue, mental health disorders such as anxiety, depression and affect interpersonal relationships. Impact of mindfulness based interventions in mental health conditions, chronic illness as well as multiple sclerosis in adults has been widely studied. Several studies have concluded that mindfulness based intervention can be beneficial in improving quality of life, mental health and physical symptoms such as fatigue in adult patients with multiple sclerosis. Current literature suggest that practice of mindfulness based techniques improve cognitive performance, attention, social skills, academic skills, emotional regulation, self-esteem, anxiety, stress and fatigue in adolescent population. There is, however, limited evidence about utilizing mindfulness based intervention in adolescents with chronic illness. The chapter describes practice of mindfulness and current research in treating symptoms of multiple sclerosis.

Chapter 11 - Pediatric multiple sclerosis is a complex disease in which the relationship between nutrition and multiple sclerosis (MS) is not well studied. Diet can play a significant role in the body's immune system and central nervous system, therefore, potentially impacting both the onset of MS or the frequency of relapse. Studies have been performed regarding the role of fats, carbohydrates, sugars, salt, vitamin D, omega-3, and lipoic acid in the disease process of MS. Further studies are needed in order to further explore the effects that nutrition has on MS. There are also limited studies specifically related to nutrition, MS, and pediatric patients. Recommendations can be made regarding lifestyle changes and regularly scheduled health maintenance visits in order to optimize patient outcomes and closely monitor nutrition status.

Chapter 12 - Multiple sclerosis is a relapsing and remitting autoimmune disease that is often more debilitating, when found in children, than when it occurs in adulthood. Though the exact etiology of MS is unknown, it is well understood that the disease process involves a complex interaction between genetic and environmental factors, of which Vitamin D level, a modifiable environmental factor, has shown a direct correlation with the progression and development of MS risk. In fact, large cohort studies, epidemiology studies, and murine models have shown that a high vitamin D level is most beneficial in MS due to its immunomodulatory effects on T cells specific to the autoimmune process. This new found data has added much promise to the treatment of MS because although one cannot change their own genetic predisposition to the disease, vitamin D level can and should be therapeutically modified for optimal management.

Chapter 13 - Major strides have been made over the last two decades in terms of understanding, identification, and subsequent treatment of multiple sclerosis. Despite the authors' increased understanding of the disease there remain many challenges. These challenges are especially poignant in pediatric MS which provides a different set of challenges in treating this population. Although there remain challenges in treatment hopefully in the future more patients will live in a disease free state or with significant reduction is disease activity. Significant strides have been made in regards to the understanding of pediatric MS and the first clinical trials are starting to look at treatment effects in these populations. This chapter will briefly review some of the emerging imaging techniques and concepts which will likely be implemented in the future treatment of pediatric MS.

SECTION ONE

In: Multiple Sclerosis in Children … ISBN: 978-1-53612-979-3
Editors: H. Omar and J. Chalkley

Chapter 1

PEDIATRIC MULTIPLE SCLEROSIS: PATHOGENESIS AND ETIOLOGY

Sharoon Qaiser**, MD
Department of Neurology, UK Healthcare, University of Kentucky, Lexington, Kentucky, US

And still they gazed, and still the wonder grew,
That one small head could carry all he knew.
(Oliver Goldsmith, The Deserted Village, 1809)

ABSTRACT

Multiple sclerosis initially thought to be disease of adults is invariably present in younger age groups as well. Most of the studies looking at pathophysiology of multiple sclerosis are based on adult patient population. Traditionally T cells were thought to be main immunological factor playing vital role in pathophysiology but recent studies suggest more complex picture involving roles of B cell, antibodies

* Correspondence: Sharoon Qaiser M.D. Fellow Physician Child Neurology. Department of Neurology. 740 S. Limestone, Lexington, KY. E-mail: sharoon.qaiser@uky.edu.

and innate immunity. Since MS is chronic inflammatory neurodegenerative disease and it's widely accepted that immune system of pediatric age group is different than adult counterparts hence a different pathophysiological model may be present. Many genetic and environmental factors play as etiological factors in MS. More research is needed to understand pathophysiology of multiple sclerosis in pediatric age group and looking into genetic and environmental etiological factors may broaden the horizon in understanding multiple sclerosis and may help in future research and treatment.

Keywords: multiple sclerosis, pediatric, pathophysiology, etiology, future research

INTRODUCTION

Multiple sclerosis is a chronic inflammatory neurodegenerative disease in which the immune system plays a pivotal role. The exact etiology of multiple sclerosis remains a mystery, despite extensive study in the triggering mechanism. The etiology of MS is likely the complex interaction between genetic factors and environmental exposures. Less is known about the pathophysiology in pediatric populations. Most of our understanding of pediatric MS is based on adult studies. Traditionally T cells were thought to be the main immunological player in regards to CNS inflammation but that view is becoming more nuanced over the last decade. The most recent evidence suggests a more complex picture which B cells, antibodies, and innate immunity all play a role in tissue damage. One of the most intriguing current debates regarding the etiology of MS is the outside-in model vs the inside-out model. The outside- in approach proposes the primary autoimmune trigger starts outside the central nervous system leading to widespread inflammation within the CNS. The latter proposes the initial event starts with the primary immune focus on the oligodendrocyte-myelin complex resulting in ongoing inflammation within the CNS [1, 2].

DISCUSSION

Although role of self-antigen as an immunological trigger is ambiguous the role of T cells plays a vital role in CNS inflammation [3]. In 2008 Banwell et al. conducted a study in which it was found that children with MS and other autoimmune diseases have exaggerated T cell response to wide variety of self-antigens. Due to lack of pediatric onset MS pathological studies, our understanding of pathogenesis is mostly based on adult studies. In adult onset MS one of the hallmark of pathophysiology is perivascular inflammatory lesions associated with demyelination and axonal injury in the white matter [3, 4]. These perivascular demyelinating lesions are further classified into four subtypes based upon the inflammation patterns. Type I has T cell/macrophage mediated immune response. Type II is mostly similar but has additional antibody mediated response. Type III and IV are different and they have little T cell mediated inflammation but have pronounced oligodendrocyte apoptosis. In case of pediatric MS, there is no sub classification. Although pathological studies are limited in pediatric MS cases but they have offered some insight in pathophysiology [3]. According to Anderson et al, many cases involve tumefactive demyelination, which is not a usual pattern in adult MS cases. In more severe phenotypes, brain biopsies showed accumulation of lymphocytes, rare B cells and macrophages in perivascular distribution. Limited biopsy studies actually showed axonal damage in normal appearing inter and intra hemispheric white matter tracts. However, it is important to note that pathological studies were mostly undertaken in more severe phenotype which may result in a biased study. There is lack of pathological studies of cortical lesions but MRI studies of pediatric MS patients show lower incidence of cortical lesions as compared to their adult counterparts [3, 4].

Multiple sclerosis does not have a pure animal model. One of the most common experimental animal model is "Experimental Autoimmune Encephalomyelitis" (EAE). In this animal model, external antigens are introduced to animal model and these highly capable antigens trigger the innate immune system. In this complicated model researchers have approximated similar key pathological pathways including demyelination, inflammation, axonal loss and gliosis. One of the key difference is that in EAE, antigen introduced is known while in human MS, it's still unclear [5]. The EAE model has not only helped us to understand pathogenesis of MS but also provided a gateway to test and develop immune modulating drugs for MS. Recent studies show vital role of gut microbe in pathogenesis of MS [6]. Human gut is a large lymphoid organ which is important site of multiple immune responses. It is already been hypothesized that patients with certain autoimmune diseases especially rheumatoid arthritis have different gut microbiome when compared to controls. In these studies, exposure to microbial agents resulted in EAE in those test animals which were disease free. In one of the recent study to look role of gut microbiome, blood and feces sample from MS patients versus controls were tested. Although there was no significant difference in the diversity of gut bacteria between two groups however according to early phase test results MS patients have increased population of Methanobrevibacter smithii and Akkermansia muciniphila and decreased population of Butyricimonas virosa. It's an interesting finding because Butyricimonas virosa produces butyrate as byproduct which is strong natural inducer of regulatory cells and it's typically decreased in MS and other auto immune diseases. Methanobrevibacter smithii is not bacteria but single cell archaeon and researches found out those with Methanobrevibacter smithii in their gut flora had unique transcription profile of their T Cells and monocytes. More research is needed to better understand role of gut flora in MS but it has been hypothesized that gut flora play a significant role in pathogenesis of MS [6].

Another aspect of understanding pathogenesis of pediatric MS is to understand pathophysiology of acute disseminated encephalomyelitis (ADEM). Acute disseminated encephalomyelitis is an acute inflammatory demyelinating disease involving encephalopathy. According to recent study [7], 15-20% confirmed pediatric MS patients had first presenting episode that was indistinguishable from ADEM. A recent study from Mayo clinic both children and adult with ADEM have evidence of limited perivascular inflammatory infiltrate but in patients with MS, these lesions involve areas beyond perivascular regions involving large areas of white matter. Another argument could be that this pathological infiltrate difference is due to age of presentation (young v/s older age group) rather that different pathological process. A small recent study done at Brigham and Women's Hospital showed that widely recognized diffusion tensor imaging changes in MS were not present in both pediatric and adult onset ADEM [8].

Since MS is inflammatory process involving central nervous system cerebrospinal fluid may provide valuable insight into pathogenesis. Historically, in adult population CSF studies include oligoclonal bands, IgG Index and cellular profile to characterize and differentiate MS from other inflammatory process. The two most commonly tested CSF inflammatory markers for MS includes IgG index and oligoclonal bands. Oligoclonal bands are bands of immunoglobulins made of IgG antibodies. Elevation of IgG levels in different inflammatory diseases of central nervous system is result of local increased synthesis of IgG. The CSF IgG index is ratio between CSF IgG and CSF albumin compared to serum IgG to serum albumin ratio. CSF index is therefore an indicator of relative amount of CSF IgG compared to serum and any increase is reflection of increased IgG production in CSF. Although it is lab specific but in most cases IgG index > 0.7 is seen in > 75% cases of MS. Although a nonspecific finding but oligoclonal bands are present in > 85% of diagnosed cases of adult MS. Due to these findings an elevated IgG index and CSF restricted oligoclonal bands are hence considered biological hallmarks of MS. If these biological markers are present at the time of initial demyelinating event, there is increase likelihood of a second attack hence differentiating it from ADEM [9].

According to Rostasy et al. [10], in one of the large study looking at CSF profiles of prepubescent children; CSF profile is different when compared to adults. CSF results were compared from eight patient groups aged between 7-29 year at onset of disease. The pediatric patients were further subdivided into two age groups with cut off of < or =11 years. CSF studies in children older than 11 years have anti myelin antibody profile similar to adults. However, children younger than 11 years of age lack the typical oligoclonal bands and only 25% of patients have raised IgG index. Other than these IgG markers, it was also found that patients < 11 years of age have higher neutrophil count as compared to >11-year-old patients. Although one possibility is age related immaturity of immune system but difference in biological immune markers in pre and post pubescent children may theoretically point towards innate immune response as opposed to adaptive response in older patients [10].

As discussed earlier, multiple studies looking at immunobiology of MS points towards simplified model of exaggerated T cell response. The initial stimulating antigen is not clear but it could be infectious or some innate antigen which causes cross reactivity with CNS antigens leading to cascade of T cell activated immune response resulting perivascular inflammation and injury. It is observed that activation of T cells is directed toward different myelin antigens (including but not limited to myelin basic protein, myelin oligodendrocyte glycoprotein and proteolipid protein etc). Although T-cell response to myelin proteins is well recognized in healthy individuals but what differentiates T cell response in case of MS is producing memory T cells phenotypes. This phenomenon could be crucial in understanding pathophysiology of MS and developing immune targeted therapies. Few studies suggested additional immune cells responsible for disease process including proinflammatory and anti-inflammatory CD4 T cells, CD8 T cells, natural killer cells and subtypes of B cells. It is not clear which process presents as initiating defect v/s immune dysregulation later in disease. Due to this concern evaluation of T cell response against myelin proteins in pediatric MS may open new horizons of better understanding of initial events which can target therapy towards prevention of disease. It is becoming increasingly clear that both cellular as well as non-cellular immune function is abnormal in MS. Cellular components implicated in MS are T lymphocytes (cytotoxic CD 8,) T-helper (CD4) type 1 and type 2, B lymphocytes monocytes, macrophages, and activated microglia. There is also wide spread dysregulation in non-cellular components including cell adhesion molecules, integrin, chemokines, and chemokine receptors.

It is widely accepted that immune system of pediatric population is different than adults. If we consider T cell immune response, thymic involution starts around puberty and results in decreased number of circulating T cells. Although number of T cells decrease post puberty but overall number of memory T cells increase resulting decreasing naïve to memory T cell ratio with aging process. Another interesting change in immunobiology in pediatric age group is that natural killer cell (NK) expression and killer cells immunoglobulin like receptors increase throughout adulthood. Recently much research emphasis is given to look into role of B cells and antibody response. One of the animal model study shows anti myelin directed antibodies which are mostly found in MS lesions are also present in autoimmune encephalomyelitis which leads to a hypothesis that may be these antibodies are related to early onset pediatric MS. There is unique opportunity to learn role of antibodies in pediatric MS as unlike their adult counterparts, antigen identification is relatively easy due to less matured epitope spread. Due to its location on the outer myelin membrane, myelin oligodendrocyte glycoprotein is an easily accessible target for antibodies. Recent studies show higher concentration of IgG antibodies against myelin oligodendrocyte glycoprotein in both pediatric MS and children with single non progressive isolated episode of ADEM. However high antibody titer is not predictor of conversion from single isolated episode of ADEM to MS. Another important myelin antigenic target is myelin basic protein which is not expressed externally but its hypothesized that there are structural abnormalities of myelin basic proteins resulting early disruption of myelin sheath and plays a role in epitope spread. The role of B cell needs to be explored more in pediatric MS to develop more specific antigen-antibody therapies [11, 12].

ETIOLOGY

The etiology of pediatric MS is promising area of research. Based on limited studies, etiological factors are divided broadly into two categories i.e., genetic susceptibility and environmental factors.

Most studies are based on findings in adult population. Highest concordance rate (27%) is found in monozygotic twins but interestingly this rate decreases significantly in dizygotic twins at 2.3%. Total incidence rate for general population is <0.1% but it increased to 2-5% for first degree relative of MS patient. The advanced whole genome mapping studies have identified variable regions of interest. Recent studies show promising association in HLA region. HLA class II haplotypes are associated with 50% genetic risk of developing MS. Given MS is inflammatory process, genome studies have also identified single nucleotide polymorphisms of interleukins especially IL-2R and IL-7R alleles, which poses risk for multiple sclerosis. Interestingly these alleles are also found in other autoimmune diseases not affecting CNS. Historically, Caucasian population has been considered high risk for MS but recently children of non-Caucasian population demonstrating higher incidence of MS as compared to their adult counterparts pointing towards environmental factors [13, 14]. Viral infections remain important environmental etiological factors in pediatric MS. Some Literature shows a many fold increased seropositivity for Epstein Barr Virus in pediatric MS cases as compared to controls of same age, independent of gender, ethnicity and genetic HLA status. But another interesting thing is a novel finding in a study [13] which showed among HLA-DRB1 positive individuals remote infection with cytomegalovirus and herpes simplex virus -1 decreased the risk of developing MS by 70% and 90% respectively but at same time if individuals are HLA-DRB1 negative HSV-1 infection increases the risk by 400% when compared to controls. These findings suggest interplay of genetics and environmental factors in determining risk of MS. Like other diseases of childhood with poor understanding of etiology and pathogenesis, link with vaccinations is been proposed but according to Mikaeloff et al. study done in French pediatric population, there is no risk associated post vaccination up to 3 years. Interesting Mikaeeloff et al. found interesting association of passive smoking and risk of MS and found twice the risk of developing MS after prolonged exposure (>10 years) of second hand smoke [15-18].

Another interesting etiological factor which may have a role in pathogenesis as well is ViT D. Multiple studies have shown decreased vitamin D levels in MS patients than controls. Vitamin D is fat soluble vitamin which has receptor expression in both neuronal tissue and immune cells [19]. A recent Mata analysis by Simpson et al. [20] showed that there is direct relation of MS incidence and latitude. Higher latitudes tend to have more prevalence of MS with the hypothesis that higher latitudes have low intensity sunlight hence decrease vitamin D. Another study further showed that childhood sun exposure and birth month (summer sunlight v/s less sun exposure) also has correlation with prevalence of MS [21]. One of the argument is that sunlight has immunosuppressive effects as studies shows UVR [21] suppressed autoimmune encephalomyelitis in animal models, so effects are related to sunlight exposure not vitamin D itself. Role of vitamin D in pathogenesis or etiological factor is unclear but it's used as a marker in disease progression. Martinelle et al. [22] showed that those presenting with single demyelinating attack, vitamin D deficiency is predictor of developing definitive MS. Despite predictive value of disease severity, risk of worsening and prevalence of MS is related to vitamin D but no randomized control trial so far has shown therapeutic advantage of vitamin D. It's important to note that few new randomized control trials looking at therapeutic effects of vitamin D are underway at this time and results are pending so role of vitamin D as effective treatment is unclear. While discussing role of Vit D, it would be relevant to discuss ethnic variation of MS. In the past it was widely believed that MS is disease which is more prevalent in Caucasian population. In recent study conducted in 2013 Langer et al. [23] conducted a retrospective cohort study of 9 million person years of multi ethnic population group and results were not consistent with popular belief. Langer at al found out that black women had highest prevalence of MS as compared to white, Hispanic or Asian individuals. Interestingly black males had similar prevalence when compared to white males. A possible hypothesis of high prevalence of MS in dark skin individual is low Vit D level. Although it's not clear why black women has highest prevalence rate of MS but it is clear now that despite historical belief white population group has no increased prevalence rate of MS.

Conclusion

In conclusion, MS is a prototypical inflammatory demyelinating disease involving central nervous system with key pathological features including inflammation, demyelination, axonal injury and glial cells reaction to injury leading to gliosis. Many studies are focused on adult population and our present understanding of pathogenesis of MS is based mostly on adult studies. More research is required to better understand pediatric MS as it may open new horizons of understanding complexity of etiological features and pathogenesis of disease and furthermore open gateway to new treatment modalities.

References

[1] Pena J, Lotze TE. Pediatric Multiple Sclerosis: Current Concepts and consensus definitions. *Autoimmune diseases* 2013;50:27-30.

[2] Krupp LB, Banwell B, et al. Consensus definitions proposed for pediatric multiple sclerosis and related disorders. *Neurology* 2007; 68(16):S7-S12.

[3] Krupp LB, Tardieu M, Amato MP, Banwell B, Chitnis T, Dale RC, et al. International Pediatric Multiple Sclerosis Study Group criteria for pediatric multiple sclerosis and immune-mediated central nervous system demyelinating disorders: revisions to the 2007 definitions. *Mult Scler*. 2013 Sep;19(10):1261-67.

[4] Anderson RC, Connolly ES Jr, Komotar RJ, Mack WJ, McKhann GM, Van Orman CB. Clinicopathological review: tumefactive demyelination in a 12-year-old girl. *Neurosurgery*. 2005 May; 56(5):1051-7.

[5] Constantinescu CS, Farooqi N, O'Brien K, Gran B. Experimental autoimmune encephalomyelitis (EAE) as a model for multiple sclerosis. *Br J Pharmacol.* 2011 Oct; 164(4): 1079–1106.

[6] Weiner HL. The gut microbiome may aid in treatment and prevention of MS. *Neurology reviews* 2015 Aug; 23(8):27-30.

[7] Banwell B., Bar-Or A, Cheung R, Kennedy J, Krupp LB, Becker DJ. Abnormal T-cell reactivities in childhood inflammatory demyelinating disease and type 1 diabetes. *Ann Neurol.* 2008 Jan;63(1):98-111.

[8] Chitnis T. Pediatric multiple sclerosis. *Neurologist.* 2006 Nov;12(6):299-310.

[9] Chabas D, Ness J, Belman A, Yeh EA, Kuntz N, Gorman MP, Strober JB, De Kouchkovsky I, McCulloch C, Chitnis T, Rodriguez M, Weinstock-Guttman B, Krupp LB, Waubant E, Younger children with MS have a distinct CSF inflammatory profile at disease onset. *Neurology.* 2010 Feb 2;74(5):399-405.

[10] Reiber H, Teut M, Pohl D, Rostasy KM, Hanefeld, F. Pediatric and adult multiple sclerosis: age related diffrences and time course of the neuroimmunological response in cerebrospinal fluid. *Mult Scler* 2009 Dec; 12:1466-80.

[11] Banwell B, Bar-Or A, Cheung R, Kennedy J, Krupp LB, Becker DJ. Abnormal T-cell reactivities in childhood inflammatory demyelinating disease and type 1 diabetes. *Ann Neurol.* 2008 Jan;63(1):98-111.

[12] Lünemann JD, Huppke P, Roberts S, Brück W, Gärtner J, Münz C. Broadened and elevated humoral immune response to EBNA1 in pediatric multiple sclerosis. *Neurology.* 2008 Sep 23;71(13):1033-5.

[13] Goodin DS. The nature of genetic susceptibility to multiple sclerosis: constraining the possibilities. *BMC Neurol.* 2016 Apr 27;16:56.

[14] Sotgiu S, Pugliatti M, Fois ML, Arru G, Sanna A, Sotgiu MA, Rosati G. Genes, environment and susceptibility to multiple sclerosis. *Neurobiol Dis.* 2004 Nov;17(2):131-43.

[15] Pohl D, Krone B, Rostasy K, Kahler E, Brunner E, Lehnert M. High seroprevalence of Epstein-Barr virus in children with multiple sclerosis. *Neurology.* 2006 Dec 12;67(11):2063-5.

[16] Waubant E, Mowry EM, Krupp L, Chitnis T, Yeh EA, Kuntz N. Common viruses associated with lower pediatric multiple sclerosis risk. *Neurology*. 2011 Jun 7;76(23):1989-95.

[17] Mikaeloff Y, Caridade G, Suissa S, Tardieu M. Hepatitis B vaccine and the risk of CNS inflammatory demyelination in childhood. *Neurology*. 2009 Mar 10;72(10):873-80.

[18] Mikaeloff Y, Caridade G, Tardieu M, Suissa S. Parental smoking at home and the risk of childhood-onset multiple sclerosis in children. *Brain*. 2007 Oct;130(Pt 10):2589-95.

[19] Alharbi FM. Update in vitamin D and multiple sclerosis. *Neurosciences* (Riyadh). 2015 Oct;20(4):329-35.

[20] Simpson S Jr, Taylor B, Blizzard L, Ponsonby AL, Pittas F, Tremlett H, Dwyer T, Gies P, van der Mei I. Higher 25-hydroxyvitamin D is associated with lower relapse risk in multiple sclerosis. *Ann Neurol.* 2010 Aug;68(2):193-20.

[21] Garcion E, Wion-Barbot N, Montero-Menei CN, Berger F, Wion D. New clues about vitamin D functions in the nervous system. *Trends Endocrinol Metab.* 2002 Apr;13(3):100-5.

[22] Martinelli V, Dalla Costa G, Colombo B, Dalla Libera D, Rubinacci A, Filippi M, Furlan R, Comi G. Vitamin D levels and risk of multiple sclerosis in patients with clinically isolated syndromes. *Mult Scler.* 2014 Feb;20(2):147-55.

[23] Langer GA, Brara SM, Beaber BE, Zhang JL. Incidence of multiple sclerosis in multiple racial and ethnic groups. *Neurology*. 2013 May 7;80(19):1734-9.

In: Multiple Sclerosis in Children … ISBN: 978-1-53612-979-3
Editors: H. Omar and J. Chalkley

Chapter 2

DIFFERENTIAL DIAGNOSIS OF MULTIPLE SCLEROSIS

Kimberly S. Jones*, MD
Department of Neurology, UK Healthcare, University of Kentucky College of Medicine, Lexington, Kentucky, US

ABSTRACT

Differentiating Multiple Sclerosis from other demyelinating disorders can be extremely challenging, but is important as these disorders can have high neurologic morbidity. With advancing treatment options, early diagnosis is more important than ever.

Keywords: multiple sclerosis, optic neuritis, transverse myelitis, acute disseminated encephalomyelitis

* Correspondence: Kimberly S. Jones, MD. Assistant Professor of Neurology, J401 Kentucky Clinic, Department of Neurology, University of Kentucky College of Medicine, Lexington, Kentucky 40536 United States. E-mail: Kimberly.Jones2@uky.edu.

Introduction

Differentiating Multiple Sclerosis from other illness can be extremely challenging, particularly because of the amount of overlap between pediatric Acquired Demyelinating Syndrome (ADS). Children can present with Acute Disseminated Encephalomyelitis (ADEM), Optic Neuritis (ON), Transverse Myelitis (TM), or other mono or polyfocal deficits. The first symptoms could represent the only attack in a monophasic disease or the initial attack in a chronic disorder, Multiple Sclerosis (MS) or Neuromyelitis Optica Sectrum Disorder (NMOSD). Exact incidence of each disorder is difficult to delineate, as they sometimes present concurrently and may vary by geographic location. Given the high potential for significant neurologic morbidity associated with these disorders and recent advances in therapeutic options, being able to identify which children are likely to have recurrence of demyelinating events is crucial.

The first step, however, is confirming the diagnosis of ADS and excluding similar disorders. The differential diagnosis for MS is quite broad, but there are a few red flags that may point you in a different direction. MS in children is the relapsing-remitting form 98% of the time, [6-10] so if a child has a progressive course, genetic, metabolic, or structural causes should be explored. Other symptoms that are unusual in pediatric MS include: evidence of peripheral nervous system involvement, end organ dysfunction, continuing systemic symptoms (fever, rash, arthralgia, weight loss), significant psychiatric symptoms, severe optic nerve pallor at presentation, or acute symptoms lasting less than 24 hours [11].

Table 1. Initial Demyelinating Attack in Children [1-5]

Optic Neuritis	29%
Transverse Myelitis	12.5%
Acute Disseminated Encephalomyelitis	25.5%
Other	33%

Table 2. Pediatric Multiple Sclerosis Differential Diagnosis

Diagnostic Category	Clinical Features
Infectious • Herpes, EBV, Enterovirus, Neuroborreliosis, • Cryptococcus • Mycoplasma, neurosyphilis	• Persistent Fever • Meningismus • Rash, petechiae • Systemic symptoms
Rheumatologic • CNS Vasculitis • Neurosarcoidosis • Bechet Syndrome • Systemic Lupus Erythematosus • Sjogren Syndrome	• Persistent headache • Systemic evidence of vasculitis • Rash • Arthralgia
Vascular Disease • Stroke • CADASIL (cerebral autosomal dominant arteriopathy with subcortical infarcts and leukoencephalopathy) • Sickle Cell Disease • Complicated Migraine	• Rapid onset of symptoms • Rapid resolution of symptoms (<24 hours) • Pain crisis • Progressive neurologic decline • Symptoms associated with headache
Metabolic/Mitochondrial • Mitochondrial Encephalomyopathy, Lactic Acidosis, Strokelike Episodes (MELAS) • Leber Hereditary Optic Neuropathy (LHON) • Leukodystrophies • Vitamin B12 or Folate Deficiency • Biotinidase deficiency	• Preexisting developmental delay or cognitive impairment • Symptoms worse with external stressor, like fever or fasting • Progressive neurologic decline • Eating disorder or Failure to Thrive
Malignancy • Glioma • CNS Lymphoma • Metastasis	• Slowly progressive symptoms • Weight loss • Prior malignancy
Paraneoplastic • Anti NMDA Receptor Encephalitis • Limbic Encephalitis	• Movement disorder • Prominent psychiatric symptoms
[11, 12]	

Acute Disseminated Encephalomyelitis in Children

Acute Disseminated Encephalomyelitis (ADEM) is an immune-mediated demyelinating CNS disease, defined clinically by acute polyfocal neurologic deficits including encephalopathy. Usually, this is thought of as a monophasic disorder that most commonly affects children. At this time, ADEM is considered to be a distinct disease from MS, but there can be overlap in the initial clinical presentation, making distinguishing between the two very difficult. There have been debates about whether encephalopathy (altered mental status, irritability, behavioral changes) should be a required part of the diagnosis of ADEM, but currently it is included to help distinguish ADEM from other acquired demyelinating diseases. ADEM is usually a monophasic disease, but a multiphasic course can occur. Updated criteria are as follows:

Table 3. Updated Criteria for ADEM

Diagnosis	Clinical Criteria
ADEM – Monophasic	(All are required): [4] • First polyfocal, clinical CNS event with presumed inflammatory demyelinating cause. • An encephalopathy that cannot be explained by fever • Brain MRI is abnormal during the acute (3 months) phase with typically diffuse, poorly demarcated large lesions involving primarily the cerebral white matter • No new clinical or MRI findings 3 months or more after onset
ADEM – Multiphasic	• ADEM followed >3 months by second ADEM episode • No further ADEM or non-ADEM demyelinating events
ADEM – Multiple Sclerosis	• ADEM followed >3 months by non-ADEM demyelinating event • New MRI lesions meeting requirements for dissemination in space
[13,14]	

Clinical Presentation

ADEM usually presents with prodromal symptoms that may include fever, malaise, nausea and vomiting, headache, somnolence or irritability. Typically, symptoms progress rapidly and peak within 2-5 days [15, 16]. However, it may be weeks or, in rare instances, months to peak symptoms. Besides encephalopathy, other neurologic symptoms commonly include seizures, hemiparesis, ataxia, optic neuritis, speech disturbance, or spinal cord findings. In 15-20% of patients, ICU admission is required, usually for respiratory failure secondary to brainstem involvement or status epilepticus [15-19]. Seizures and fever are symptoms that may be most specific for ADEM, as opposed to MS. Outcomes are favorable, with the majority of children reported to make a full recovery, usually within weeks [15, 19]. Mortality rates, however, are still reported to be between 1-3% [17, 18]. There are some recent studies showing long term cognitive and behavior deficits as well, especially if ADEM occurs before 5 years of age [21, 22].

MRI findings in ADEM – T2 and FLAIR images typically show bilateral large and poorly demarcated hyperintense lesions. They are multifocal and often involve the deep gray structures or the brainstem. Spinal cord lesions are reported in up to ¼ of patients and are commonly longitudinally extensive (longer than 3 vertebral segments) [13, 16]. Lesions do not usually enhance with gadolinium administration. However, as many as 30% of patients will have a few of the small lesions that do [16]. Though there are a lot of similarities between MR images of patients with ADEM and MS, recent studies show that there are some specific characteristics that help distinguish the two. Specifically, absence of periventricular lesions points towards ADEM. The presence of well-defined lesions perpendicular to the ventricle (Dawson's fingers) and T1 hypointense lesions have the highest predictive value in distinguishing children who will develop MS [24, 25]. By the definition above, ADEM is not associated with new lesions after 3 months of onset and most patients have been found to have complete or near complete resolution of lesions on follow up imaging [19]. At this time, there are no specific imaging guidelines, but reimaging the child after 3 months may have an important role in ruling out disease progression or evidence of another diagnosis.

Transverse Myelitis in Children

Acute transverse myelitis (ATM) makes up about 20% of ADS in children on their first attack. It differs from ADEM in that it is more common in adults (80%) [26,27] and has a much higher rate of poor recovery. Clinically, over half of children report a prodromal illness within the month prior to symptom onset [2, 27-31]. Children commonly present with back pain, sometimes quite severe (60%) [2, 31]. Then, they develop motor and sensory symptoms, as well as bowel and bladder dysfunction. Symptoms usually peak in about 5-6 days [27, 31, 32] bladder and sensory symptoms take the longest to resolve [31]. Sensory symptoms can be positive (tinging, burning, Lhermittes, etc) or negative (numbness). Children do not always have complete paraparesis, symptoms can be asymmetric or patchy. On examination, patients should have a spinal sensory level, but this can be difficult to illicit from small children. Involvement of the posterior columns can present as an ataxic gait or fine motor deficits. Initially, children may have symptoms of spinal shock with flaccid weakness and hyporeflexia. This may take up to 12 weeks to resolve, with subsequent development of spasticity and hyerreflexia. During this recovery phase, a child has increased risk of developing autonomic dysreflexia with bradycardia and hypotension.

Table 4. Transverse Myelitis Consortium Working Group Criteria

Sensory, motor, or autonomic dysfunction attributable to the spinal cord
Bilateral involvement, may be asymmetric
Presence of a sensory level
Progression to nadir 4 hours to 21 days
Absence of symptoms attributable to acquired brain demyelinating syndrome
Exclusion of compressive or infectious etiology

Table 5. Definite Transverse Myelitis includes 1 of

CSF pleocytosis >10 leukocytes/mm^3
Elevated IgG index or presence of intrathecal oligoclonal bands
MRI spinal gadolinium enhancement

MRI of the spinal cord typically shows T2 hyerintense lesions that are centrally located. Lesions may be contiguous or patchy. Children mostly have longitudinally extensive TM (LETM, defined as greater than vertebral 3 segments), reports range from 66-85% [33, 34]. The lesions usually enhance with gadolinium, but this is not a requirement for the diagnosis. Up to 1/3 of TM lesions in children are described to have T1 hypointensity as well [27, 32, 34].

Outcome

Prognosis is better in children than adults, with half making a full recovery by 2 years. However, there can be considerable morbidity in those who do not fully recover with 10-20% never regaining any mobility or bladder function. The largest study designed to identify predictive factors for relapse included 95 patients with a median follow-up of 1.4 years. Sixteen patients had a subsequent attack (17%). Thirteen had relapses and brain MRI lesions that met the criteria for MS [33]. Three developed NMO (all were aquaporin-4 ab positive). Notably, of the 20 patients in the monophasic TM category who were screened for aquaporin-4 antibodies, 2 others were positive as well [33]. This study concluded that 2 risk factors for relapse include abnormal brain MRI and female gender.

Demyelinating Optic Neuritis in Children

Approximately 30% of children will present with ON as the initial demyelinating syndrome. It occurs as an isolated event in most children, but can be associated with multifocal demyelinating syndromes ADEM,

MS, Chronic relapsing inflammatory optic neuropathy (CRION), and NMO. Differentiating between these has significant treatment and prognostic implications. Clinical presentation in children is often different than adults, and is commonly associated with profound vision loss. Children under the age of 10 present with bilateral optic neuritis 72% of the time, whereas ON is unilateral in 70% of children > 10 years of age [35, 36]. Also, ON in children tends to be more anterior than typical ON in adults [37, 39]. Clinically, children have decreased visual acuity, dyschromatopsia (particularly with red color desaturation), and visual field defects. Over 60% of children have visual acuity of 20/200 or worse [47, 41]. Pain with eye movement is taught as a cardinal feature, but is reported inconsistently and may be difficult for younger children to distinguish from headache, which is also a common symptom [41]. Patients have relative afferent pupillary defect and funduscopic exam acutely shows papillitis in approximately half of children with ON [42]. Symptoms develop quickly and usually peak within a few days.

MRI of head and orbits should be obtained. Typical findings with ON include hyperintense T2 signal and thickening of the optic nerve with post-contrast enhancement. Findings of T2 hyerintense lesions in other areas of the brain are associated with an increased risk of developing MS. Longitudinally extensive lesions of the optic nerve may be associated with NMO, but further studies need to be done to confirm this finding [43,44].

Visual Evoked Potentials have prolonged P100 latencies. In children with unilateral ON, abnormal VEP in the unaffected eye may suggest an increased risk of MS [45].

Outcome

Recovery of visual acuity usually occurs in about three weeks from symptom onset, but can take longer than a year, particularly in children [38, 46]. Prognosis is good with isolated demyelinating ON, with 58-96% returning to better than 20/40 visual acuity [40, 41, 47, 48].

Table 6. International Panel on NMO Diagnostic Criteria, revised 2014 [52]

NMO-IgG seropositive and at least one of the following *OR* seronegative and at least 2 of the following:
Optic Neuritis
Transverse Myelitis (LETM if sero negative for NMO IgG)
Area Postrema Syndrome
Acute Brainstem Syndrome
Narcolepsy or Diencephalic Syndrome
Cerebral Syndrome with NMO-typical brain lesions

NMO in Children

Neuromyelitis Optica (NMO) disorder is traditionally thought of as an inflammatory disease with repeated attacks of optic neuritis and longitudinally extensive transverse myelitis (LETM). It is rare compared to MS and only 4% of NMO cases are reported to have pediatric onset [49-51]. Pathogenic antibodies, NMO-IgG, have been discovered. They are directed against aquaporin-4, a water channel found in astrocytes that form the blood brain barrier that is heavily concentrated in areas commonly affected in NMO patients. Since the discovery of the NMO-IgG, there has been recognition of a spectrum in NMO (NMOSD) that can involve other areas of the nervous system, like the dorsal medulla or hypothalamus. Based on these findings, diagnostic criteria have been revised and are summarized in the table above. They need further validation in children.

Clinical Feature

The most common presenting features of NMO in children were visual, motor, and constitutional (fever, vomiting, seizures), with lesions seen in the optic nerves, spinal cord, and brainstem. About half of children have episodic symptoms that localize outside of the optic nerves or spinal cord [51, 53]. Optic neuritis can be unilateral or bilateral. Vision loss may be more severe in NMO, but otherwise cannot be clinically distinguished from MS. Spinal cord symptoms can be severe, with paresis and sensory loss, as well as bowel and bladder dysfunction. Neuropathic pain and paroxysmal tonic muscle spasms can be debilitating. Symptoms that may point toward NMO, as opposed to the other demyelinating disorders, include intractable hiccups or vomiting and narcolepsy.

MRI Findings

Optic nerve T2 hyperintensities and swelling, with gadolinium enhancement on T1 weighted sequences are similar to those seen in MS. Children with NMO more commonly have bilateral optic nerve lesions that tend to be more posterior, often involving the optic chiasm. Spinal cord lesions of NMO are more frequent in the cervical and upper thoracic cord. They have T2 hyperintense signal with hypointense signal on T1 weighted images, typically involving the central gray matter. Lesions involving more than 3 vertebral segments (LETM) are more specific for NMO in adults. However, in children, this is commonly seen with ADEM, MS, and monophasic TM. Children with NMO can have subcortical or deep white matter T2 hyperintensities that are indistinguishable from MS. However, lesions in the periependymal regions are more specific for NMO. LETM can extend up into dorsal medulla surrounding the 4th ventricle and include the area postrema. When associated with intractable vomiting, this is highly specific for NMO. Lesions of the thalamus and hypothalamus, around the 3rd ventricle, can lead to diencephalon syndrome with significant hormone imbalance or narcolepsy. Lesions around the lateral ventricles are common, as well. However, unlike MS, they tend to be confluent and follow the ependymal lining [53].

Outcome

Data is limited, but a recent study comparing NMO to other demyelinating disorders in children found that the number of attacks and clinical disability at 2 years was higher in NMO than MS. That being said, it also showed that the average time to diagnosis was close to 1 year, so treatment delay may be a contributing factor [49].

CONCLUSION

With advancing treatment options for demyelinating disorders, it is critical to diagnosis chronic recurring disease as soon as possible. However, in children, this can be extremely difficult given the high rate of Acute Disseminated Enephalomyelitis and other monophasic demyelinating syndromes relative to adults. A typical bout of ADEM can be the initial presentation in Multiple Sclerosis or Neuromyelitis Optic Spectrum Disorder, complicating the picture even further. Even diagnosing ADEM can be difficult, given the wide range of other infectious and non-infectious disorders that may present with a similar clinical picture (see Table 2).

The 2010 McDonald criteria for diagnosing MS can be reliably applied to children down to age 12. There is some recent data to suggest that children even younger than 12 who present with Clinically Isolated Syndrome (without encephalopathy) and meet the criteria for dissemination in space and time are likely to be confirmed to have multiple sclerosis within 2 years. However, at this point in time, if a child presents with encephalopathy, there is no reliable way to confirm a diagnosis of multiple sclerosis during the first attack. A positive serum NMO-IgG, along with typical clinical and MRI features of neuromyelitis optic spectrum disorder would meet diagnostic criteria, though further study is needed to validate these criteria in children. Reevaluating children 3 or more months after a bout of ADEM, may reveal new lesions that would point to a diagnosis of MS. If symptoms are more concerning for NMO, repeating serum NMO-IgG levels may be useful, as there are reports of children not becoming seropositive until as long as 39 months after symptom onset. More data is needed to determine specific guidelines for evaluating children with acute demyelination. Given the cumulative morbidity of recurrent attacks, diligent follow up leading to earlier diagnosis and treatment initiation should be a focus moving forward.

References

[1] Brenton JN, Banwell BL. Therapeutic approach to the management of pediatric demyelinating disease: Multiple sclerosis and acute disseminated encephalomyelitis. *Neurotherapeutics.* 2016 Jan;13(1):84-95.

[2] Banwell B1, Kennedy J, Sadovnick D, Arnold DL, Magalhaes S, Wambera K, et al. Incidence of acquired demyelination of CNS in Canadian children. *Neurology*. 2009 Jan 20;72(3):232-9.

[3] Langer-Gould A, Zhang JL, Chung J, Yeung Y, Waubant E, Yao J. Incidence of acquired CNS demyelinating syndromes in a multi-ethnic cohort of children. *Neurology.* 2011 Sep 20;77(12):1143-8.

[4] Ketelslegers IA, Catsman-Berrevoets CE, Neuteboom RF, Boon M, van Dijk KG, Eikelenboom MJ, et al. Incidence of acquired demyelinating syndromes of the CNS in Dutch children: a nationwide study. *J Neurol.* 2012 Sep;259(9):1929-35.

[5] Absoud M, Lim MJ, Chong WK, De Goede CG, Foster K, Gunny R, et al. Paediatric acquired demyelinating syndromes: incidence, clinical, and magnetic resonance imaging features. *Mult Scler.* 2013 Jan 19(1):76-86.

[6] Chou IJ, Wang HS, Whitehouse WP, Constantinescu CS. Paediatric Multiple Sclerosis: Update on diagnostic criteria, imaging, histopathology and treatment choices. *Curr Neurol Neurosci Rep.* 2016 Jul;16(7):68.

[7] Renoux C, Vukusic S, Mikaeloff Y, Edan G, Clanet M, Dubois B, et al. Natural history of multiple sclerosis with childhood onset. *N Engl J Med* 2007;356(25):2603-13.

[8] Harding KE, Liang K, Cossburn MD, Ingram G, Hirst CL, Pickersgill TP, et al. Long-term outcome of paediatric-onset multiple sclerosis: a population-based study. *J Neurol Neurosurg Psychiatry* 2013;84(2):141-7.

[9] Ghezzi A, Deplano V, Faroni J, Grasso MG, Liguori M, Marrosu G, et al. Multiple sclerosis in childhood: clinical features of 149 cases. *Mult Scler* 1997;3(1):43-6.

[10] Duquette P, Murray TJ, Pleines J, Ebers GC, Sadovnick D, Weldon P, et al. Multiple sclerosis in childhood: clinical profile in 125 patients. *J Pediatr* 1987;111(3):359-63.

[11] Narula S, Banwell B. Pediatric Demyelination. *Continuum* 2016;22(3):897-915.

[12] Jancic J, Nikolic B, Ivancevic N, Djuric V, Zaletel I, Stevanovic D, et al. Multiple sclerosis in pediatrics: current concepts and treatment options. *Neurol Ther.* 2016 Dec 5(2):131-43.

[13] Tardieu M, Banwell B, Wolinsky JS, Pohl D, Krupp LB. Consensus definitions for pediatric MS and other demyelinating disorders in childhood. *Neurology* 2016;87 (suppl 2):S8-S11.

[14] Wassmer E, Chitnis T, Pohl D, et al. International Pediatric MS Study Group Global Members Symposium report. *Neurology* 2016;87 (suppl 2):S110-15.

[15] Pohl D, Gulay A, Van Haran K, Kornberg AJ, Lucchinetti CF, Tenembaum S, et al. Acute disseminated encephalomyelitis: Updates on an inflammatory CNS syndrome. *Neurology* 2016;87 (suppl 2):S38-45.

[16] Tenembaum S, Chamoles N, Fejerman N. Acute disseminated encephalomyelitis: A long term follow-up study of 84 pediatric patients. *Neurology* 2002;59:1224-31.

[17] Absoud M, Parslow RC, Wassmer E, et al. Severe acute disseminated encephalomyelitis: a paediatric intensive care population-based study. *Mult Scler* 2011;17:1258-61.

[18] Ketelslegers IA, Visser IE, Neuteboom RF, Boon M, Catsman-Berrevoets CE, Hintzen RQ. Disease course and outcome of acute disseminated encephalomyelitis is more severe in adults than in children. *Mult Scler* 2011;17:411-88.

[19] Tenembaum S, Chitnis T, Ness J, Hahn JS, Acute disseminated encephalomyelitis. *Neurology* 2007;68 (suppl 2):S23-S26.

[20] Tenembaum SN. Acute disseminated encephalomyelitis. *Handb Clin Neurol* 2013;112:1253-62.

[21] Jacobs RK, Anderson VA, Neale JL, Shield LK, Kornberg AJ. Neuropsychological outcome after acute disseminated encephalomyelitis: impact of age at illness onset. *Pediatr Neurol* 2004;31:191-7.

[22] Suppiej A, Cainelli E, Casara G, Cappellari A, Nosadini M, Sartori S. Long-term neurocognitive outcome and quality of life in pediatric acute disseminated encephalomyelitis. *Pediatr Neurol* 2014;50:363-7.

[23] Murthy SN, Faden HS, Cohen ME, Bakshi R. Acute disseminated encephalomyelitis in children. *Pediatrics* 2002;110(2 pt 1):E21.

[24] Banwell B, Ghezzi A, Bar-Or A, et al. Multiple sclerosis in children: clinical diagnosis, therapeutic strategies, and future directions. *Lancet Neurol* 2007;6(10):887-902.

[25] Chitnis T, Glanz B, Jaffin S, Healy B. Demographics of pediatric-onset multiple sclerosis in an MS center population from Northeastern United States. *Mult Scler* 2009;15(5):627-31.

[26] Absoud M, Greenberg BM, Lim M, Lotze T, Thomas T, Deiva K. Pediatric transverse myelitis. *Neurology* 2016;87(suppl 2):S46-S52.

[27] Pidcock FS, Krishnan C, Crawford TO, Salorio CF, Trovato M, Kerr DA. Acute transverse myelitis in childhood: center-based analysis of 47 cases. *Neurology* 2007;68:1474-80.

[28] Wolf VL, Lupo PJ, Lotze TE. Pediatric acute transverse myelitis: overview and differential diagnosis. *J Child Neurol* 2012;(11):1426-36.

[29] Kerr DA, Ayetey H. Immunopathogenesis of acute transverse myelitis. *Curr Opin Neurol* 2002;15(3):339-47.

[30] Miyazawa R, Ikeuchi Y, Tomomasa T, Ushiku H, Ogawa T, Morikawa A. Determinants of prognosis of acute transverse myelitis in children. *Pediatr Int* 2003; 45:512-6.

[31] Thomas T, Branson HM, Verhey LH, et al. The demographic, clinical, and magnetic resonance imaging (MRI) features of transverse myelitis in children. *J Child Neurol* 2012;27(1):11-21.

[32] De Goede CG, Holmes EM, Pike MG. Acquired transverse myelopathy in children in the United Kingdom: a 2 year prospective study. *Eur J Paediat Neurol* 2010; 14:479-87.

[33] Deiva K, Absoud M, Hemingway C, et al. Acute idiopathic transverse myelitis in children: early predictors of relapse and disability. *Neurology* 2015;84:341-9.

[34] Alper G, Petropoulou KA, Fitz CR, Kim Y. Idiopathic acute transverse myelitis in children: an analysis and discussion of MRI findings. *Mult Scler* 2011;17:74-80.

[35] Yeh EA, Graves JS, Benson LA, Wassmer E, Waldman A. Pediatric optic neuritis. *Neurology* 2016;87(suppl 2):S53-S58.

[36] Waldman AT, Stull LB, Galetta SL, Balcer LJ, Liu GL. Pediatric optic neuritis and risk of multiple sclerosis: meta-analysis of observational studies. *J AAPOS* 2011;15:441-6.

[37] Collinge JE, Sprunger DT. Update in pediatric optic neuritis. *Curr Opin Ophthalmol* 2013;24:448-52.

[38] El-Dairi MA, Ghasia F, Bhatti MT. Pediatric optic neuritis. *Int Ophthalmol Clin* 2012;52:29-49.

[39] Albert DM, Jakobiec FA, Miller JW, Azar DT. Optic neuritis. In: Gabbedy RJ, Knowles Z, editors. *Principles and practice of ophthalmology,* 3rd ed. North America: Elsevier Saunders; 2008:3871-85.

[40] Bonhomme GR, Waldman AT, Balcer LJ, Daniels AB, Tennekoon GI, Forman S, et al. Pediatric optic neuritis: brain MRI abnormalities and risk of multiple sclerosis. *Neurology* 2009;72:232-9.

[41] Wiljeto M, Shroff M, Buncic JR, Kennedy J, Goia C, Banwell B. The clinical features, MRI findings, and outcome of optic neuritis in children. *Neurology* 2006;67:258-62.

[42] Morales DS, Siatkowski RM, Howard CW, Warman R. Optic neuritis in children. *J Pediatr Ophthalmol Strabismus* 2000;37:254-9.

[43] Ramanathan S, Prelog K, Barnes EH, Tantsis EM, Reddel SW, Henderson AP, et al. Radiological differentiation of optic neuritis with myelin oligodendrocyte glycoprotein antibodies, aquaporin-4 antibodies, and multiple sclerosis. *Mult Scler.* 2016 Apr 22(4):470-82.

[44] Graves J, Kraus V, Soares BP, Hess CP, Waubant E. Longitudinally extensive optic neuritis in pediatric patients. *J Child Neurol* 2015;30:120-3.

[45] Pohl D, Rostasy K, Treiber-Held S, Brockman K, Gartner J, Hanefeld F. Pediatric multiple sclerosis: detection of clinically silent lesions by multimodal evoked potentials. *J Pediatr* 2006;149:125-7.

[46] Lucchinetti CF, Kiers L, O'Duffy A, Gomez MR, Cross S, Leavitt JA, et al. Risk factors for developing multiple sclerosis after childhood optic neuritis. *Neurology.* 1997 Nov 49(5):1413-8.

[47] Malik MT, Healy BC, Benson LA, Kivisakk P, Musallam A, Weiner HL, et al. Factors associated with recovery from acute optic neuritis in patients with multiple sclerosis. *Neurology*. 2014 Jun 17;82(24):2173-9.

[48] Absoud M, Cummins C, Desai N, Gika A, McSweeney N, Munot P, et al. Childhood optic neuritis clinical features and outcome. *Arch Dis Child.* 2011 Sep;96(9):860-2.

[49] Chitnis T, Ness J, Krupp L, Waubant E, et al. Clinical features of neuromyelitis optica in children: US Network of Pediatric MS Centers report. *Neurology* 2016;86:245-52.

[50] Quek AM, McKeon A, Lennon VA, Mandrekar JN, Iorio R, Jiao Y, et al. Effects of age and sex on aquaporin-4 autoimmunity in children. *Arch Neurology* 2012;69:1039-43.

[51] McKeon A, Lennon VA, Lotze T, Tenenbaum S, Ness JM, Rensel M, et al. CNS aquaporin-4 autoimmunity in children. *Neurology.* 2008 Jul 8;71(2):93-100.

[52] Wingerchuk DM, Banwell B, Bennett JL, Cabre P, Carroll W, Chitnis T, et al. International consensus diagnostic criteria for neuromyelitis optica spectrum disorders. *Neurology.* 2015 Jul 14;85(2):177-89.

[53] Kim HJ, Paul F, Lana-Peixoto MA, Tenembaum S, Asgari N, Palace J, et al. MRI Characteristics of neuromyelitis optica spectrum disorder: An international update. *Neurology.* 2015 Mar 17;84(11):1165-73.

In: Multiple Sclerosis in Children … ISBN: 978-1-53612-979-3
Editors: H. Omar and J. Chalkley

Chapter 3

CLINICAL MANIFESTATIONS OF PEDIATRIC-ONSET MULTIPLE SCLEROSIS

Valeria I. Naranjo, MD and Donita D. Lightner, MD*
Department of Neurology, UK Healthcare, University of Kentucky College of Medicine, Lexington, Kentucky, US

ABSTRACT

Pediatric multiple sclerosis is very uncommon and clinical presentations, particularly in pre-adolescent patients, can vary dramatically as compared to post adolescent or adult manifestations of disease. The purpose of this chapter is to compare and contrast these differences by our clinical experience/patient vignettes and review the literature.

Keywords: pediatric multiple sclerosis, manifestations of multiple sclerosis, acute disseminated encephalomyelitis, optic neuritis, encephalitis

---

* Corresponding author: Donita D. Lightner, MD. Assistant Professor of Neurology, J422 Kentucky Clinic, Department of Neurology, University of Kentucky College of Medicine, Lexington, Kentucky 40536 United States. E-mail: donita.lightner@uky.edu.

Introduction

As in adult multiple sclerosis (MS), clinical attacks in pediatric MS are disseminated in time and space, which helps differentiate the condition from other demyelinating diseases. The vast majority of pediatric MS follows a relapsing-remitting course [1-3], with evolution of symptoms and symptom resolution for months to years. Due to the temporal nature of the diagnosis and difficulties in obtaining accurate histories from younger children, diagnosing multiple sclerosis in children is often challenging.

Case Vignettes

Here are two examples of children diagnosed with MS. Note the differences between the two cases.

Case 1

SM, a previously-healthy 14-year-old Caucasian female, presented to the emergency department with a recent history of migrating weakness and numbness. The first episode lasted for a total of two weeks and involved 1-2 day periods of waxing-and-waning numbness involving her face, right arm, and left leg. Two weeks later she experienced weakness and numbness of her upper and lower extremities at the same time, which prompted her to see a neurologist who ordered magnetic resonance imaging (MRI). Before the study could be performed, she developed worsening numbness and weakness of her upper right extremity and bilateral lower extremities, which led her to present to the emergency room. She was admitted to the hospital and found to have four demyelinating lesions on MRI. A diagnosis of MS was made, and she was started on intravenous methylprednisolone. After 5 days, she was sent home on daily glatiramer. She remained symptom-free for four months, then developed left sided facial numbness and left eye pain, followed by diplopia. She was admitted again and found to have new demyelinating lesions on MRI.

At two years from her diagnosis, SM has been without major relapse for over a year. She is on disease-modifying therapy, and current issues include persistent fatigue and subjective difficulties with balance. She now suffers from depression, and was started on medication for it. Recent MRI demonstrated stable white matter lesions.

Case 2

FS, a three-year-six-month old Caucasian girl, was admitted to the hospital for evaluation due to a three-day history of frequent falls, dragging her left foot, and decreased use of her left hand. Over the year prior to presentation, FS saw her pediatrician multiple times; first for stuttering and rash after a tick bite, and several months later for crossed eyes. She was seen by ophthalmology and her parents were told she would "grow out of it." Three weeks prior to her hospital admission, she was acting "like a baby" to her mom, and developed diurnal enuresis. During her initial hospitalization, MRI revealed multiple areas of T2 hyper intensity. Infectious disease specialist was consulted due to previous concerns for tick-borne illness and an extensive infectious evaluation was negative. She was diagnosed with acute disseminated encephalomyelitis (ADEM) at the time. Lumbar puncture was performed, but her cerebrospinal fluid (CSF) was unremarkable, with normal IgG and no oligoclonal bands. MS profile showed elevated myelin basic protein. She was started on intravenous steroids and sent home with a steroid taper. She returned to her normal state of health until two months after discharge, when she developed staring spells, fever, slurred speech and inability to follow directions. She was readmitted, and found to have new lesions on MRI. She again received steroids and was sent home on steroid taper, with what was thought to be a progression or recurrence of ADEM or possible MS. She again returned to baseline, and one month later developed behavioral changes, right leg weakness, hand tremors, and inward-deviation of her right eye. MRI then showed an increased number of white matter lesions. It was after multiple attacks, that CSF oligoclonal bands became positive. She was hospitalized and after consultation with pediatric neuroimmunologic specialists she was diagnosed with childhood MS, and started on monthly intravenous immunoglobulin (IVIG). After she continued to have multiple relapses despite IVIG therapy, a brain biopsy was performed and demonstrated findings consistent with MS or ADEM.

Over the next 3 years, FS had numerous hospitalizations for relapses with similar symptoms as described above. She was ultimately started on disease-modifying antirheumatic drugs (DMARD), but continues to experience periodic relapses.

Clinical Presentation

As demonstrated by the clinical vignettes, the presentation of pediatric multiple sclerosis (MS) varies greatly from patient to patient. Up to 5% of all cases of MS are thought to occur before the age of 18, with about 17% of those before the age of 12, and with a varying female-to-male ratio depending on age of presentation. Female to male preponderance appears to be higher in adolescent and adult-onset MS (rate of 1.5-3 to 1) [2, 4-9].

Symptoms frequently depend upon the age of the child, although initial bouts usually involve afferent structures of the central nervous system [10]. The presentation of pediatric and adolescent multiple sclerosis is highly variable in type and severity and patients can present initially with almost any CNS sign or symptom, from motor and sensory symptoms, altered mental status or encephalopathy, constitutional, cognitive and school problems, and even mood and behavioral changes [11, 21].

Ultimately, signs and symptoms depend on the localization of the defect or the area of damage. Whereas adult MS is often initially monosymptomatic, pediatric MS is frequently polysymptomatic [4, 12-14].

Below are general signs and symptoms that may be observed, dependent upon the localization of affected areas:

Motor symptoms involve motor weakness, stiffness or spasticity, hemiparesis or incontinence. Motor symptoms are also the most likely to persist after an attack, which may involve weakness or loss of muscle strength and dexterity.

Problems with coordination or balance include ataxia, which occurs in just over 50% of patients [15].

Sensory symptoms, including numbness or tingling of extremities, as well as headaches or other kinds of pain, can be present. Visual symptoms commonly include blurred or double vision, or temporary loss of sight in one eye or both. Diplopia represents brainstem dysfunction (as in internuclear ophthalmoplegia), whereas vision loss often indicates optic neuritis.

Constitutional symptoms are a more defining characteristic of pediatric MS than adult-onset MS, and include fever (22%) and fatigue (up to 40% of patients with activity-limiting fatigue [15], described as an overwhelming sense of tiredness, making physical or mental activity difficult).

Cognitive functioning difficulties are common in pediatric MS, found in about 30% to 50% of children with MS [16-19], although due to preserved verbal fluency in most patients it is frequently unrecognized. Complex attention (shifting attention from one idea to another), visuomotor integration, receptive language, verbal and visual memory, and executive function problems have been most commonly described. Social cognition, such as facial recognition of affective state and knowledge of others has been reported [15, 16]. As in adults with MS, cognitive problems can be detected from the early stages of the disease, unrelated to the level of physical disability, and can have a negative impact on lifestyle, school achievements, and overall quality of life [19].

Mood disturbances, in particular depressive symptoms and behavioral problems, including anxiety, depression, mood swings or irritability, are also increasingly recognized in children with MS [19, 20].

Current data highlights significant differences between adolescent and pre-adolescent MS. Whereas adolescents tend to mirror the adult form of the disease, pre-adolescents often present with atypical features (e.g., polysymptomatic presentations, encephalopathy, constitutional symptoms, seizures, etc.) [1, 15, 21]. Therefore, we will continue by discussing the adult-similar adolescent form, followed by the pre-adolescent form of MS.

Adolescent Multiple Sclerosis

Initial features that are predictive of MS include older age and female sex (in adolescent and adult-onset MS) and presence of polyfocal signs [12, 22, 23]. Like adults, post-pubertal patients predominantly present with optic neuritis, transverse myelitis and sensory symptoms, suggesting spinal cord involvement [3, 4, 6].

In adolescents, one large study revealed the most common symptoms were: sensory (54%), motor (45%), vision (39%), coordination (32%), constitutional (29%), bowel-bladder (8%), encephalopathy (2%) [4]. Adolescents are more likely to have monosymptomatic or monofocal presentations [1]. Studies suggest that the initial symptom pattern can prevail over the first 2 years of disease [24].

Pre-Adolescent Multiple Sclerosis

In general, younger children have more atypical presentations. Preceding events like fever or infections, as well as trauma or falls are more readily identifiable in younger children as compared to adolescents, suggesting MS as an acute postinfectious inflammatory disorder [4, 6, 7].

Pre-pubertal patients were more likely to have a polysymptomatic severe first attack with motor and brainstem involvement, sphincter dysfunction, cognitive disturbances and milder residual neurological sequelae after the first episode compared to older patients and adults [24, 33].

Sensory symptoms are reported less commonly in this population, which may be partially attributable to the challenges of accurate symptom reporting in children.

Conversely, encephalopathy, seizures, and ataxia or motor and coordination problems are more common in young children [4]. Seizures, which are rarely seen in adolescent and adult MS, are more common in the polysymptomatic presentation of younger children and seen in about 5% of cases [1, 15].

In one large study of pediatric MS4, the relative frequency of initial symptoms children less than 12 years of age was: motor (56%), coordination (50%), vision (48%), constitutional (42%), sensory (20%), encephalopathy (16%), bowel-bladder symptoms (13%). Seizures occur in about 5% of children, more common in children younger than 10 years of age [15].

Progression and Relapse Rate

Compared to adult MS, children and adolescents with MS have slower progression of the disease, particularly during the early stages, suggesting greater plasticity in the younger nervous system [25, 26]. A study estimated that patients with childhood-onset disease take approximately 10 years longer to reach secondary progression and irreversible disability, but reached these landmarks at an age approximately 10 years younger ($P < 0.001$) [2]. This age group experiences a higher relapse rate, but also most pediatric patients have complete recovery after their first attacks. However, this population also displays permanent disability at an earlier age [1, 12].

The disease course of MS can be divided into a relapsing-remitting phase, with predominance of inflammatory mechanisms, and a progressive phase, with predominant neurodegenerative mechanisms. Acute relapses are the clinical hallmark of the inflammatory phase of MS [25]. Pediatric MS appears to be overall a more inflammatory disease than adult MS, with more frequent relapses and lesion accrual on MRI. This fact may be related to different immune activation or levels of cells and cytokines in the CNS of pediatric patients [13, 18, 27].

There are age group-specific differences as well, for instance adolescents generally have a second clinical attack within 12 months after the first event, whereas the younger children have a greater time interval between the first and second attacks.

The ultimate goal of therapy in MS is to prevent these relapses and ultimately disability accrual. The concept of non-evident disease activity, measured by absence of clinical and MRI disease is considered the overall goal for treatment. This has not yet been systematically evaluated in pediatric MS, but data from the adult counterparts suggests that despite advances in therapy, this is achieved in just close to 50% of adults with MS followed for 2 years in therapeutic trials, while longitudinal data have shown that only 7% of adult patients with MS have no evidence of disease activity at 7 years of follow-up [18].

PROGNOSIS

The prognosis often depends upon the severity and location of initial and subsequent attacks, and the timing and frequency of relapses. Relapsing and remitting disease has been found to have the most favorable prognosis [6]. Optic neuritis in childhood is thought to be more likely bilateral and less likely to lead to MS versus in adults [28, 29]. Optic neuritis also often portends a more benign prognosis [30].

Listed below are poor prognostic factors for severity of clinical disease:

- Extremely early onset of MS; e.g., in the toddler years [7].
- A short interval (less than 1 year) between the first 2 demyelinating episodes is associated with an increased risk of having a third attack or scoring higher on the Expanded Disability Status Scale (EDSS).
- An incomplete recovery after the first attack is associated with a greater risk of having additional attacks with incomplete recovery, increasing the risk of cumulative disability over time.

- Brainstem involvement at onset portends a poor prognosis, with a risk of secondary progressive disease in the future more than 5 times higher than in children whose initial attack affects other brain regions [1, 12, 30].
- The frequency of relapses, especially during the first 5 years of the disease, and the duration of the first and the second remission appear to correlate with the risk of early secondary progressive form and permanent disability, as also seen in the adult counterpart [12, 31].
- Among patients with progressive disease, those with frequent relapses have the most unfavorable outlook, with a statistically significant correlation between rate of relapses and rate of progression [6].

LONG-TERM EFFECTS

Pediatric MS carries with it a significant burden of morbidity and variable levels of disability. To help gauge disability, the Expanded Disability Status Scale (EDSS) is commonly used. The clinical presentation of the disability depends upon the specific neurologic tract involvement, which EDSS describes in terms of "functional system." Functional systems include mental/cerebral, bowel and bladder, pyramidal (motor), brainstem, visual, cerebellar and sensory.

Children generally score an EDSS of 3.00 +/- 1.57 (a score of 3 indicates moderate disability while still ambulatory) at 5 years out from disease diagnosis [30], and one study reported that 8 years from diagnosis over 50% of patients had EDSS of > = 4 (severe disability while able to ambulate 500m) [32]. Another study estimated the median time from onset to secondary progression to be 28 years, and the median age at conversion to secondary progression was 41 years [2].

Conclusion

- The vast majority of pediatric MS follows a relapsing-remitting course [1-3]
- In younger individuals with pediatric MS, the female: male ratio is lower. This is in contrast with a female preponderance after puberty, as also seen in adults [2, 4-9].
- They can present with almost any CNS sign or symptom (motor, sensory symptoms, encephalopathy, constitutional, cognitive, mood and behavioral) [11, 18, 21].
- A polyfocal presentation is more common in the younger patients.
- Initial attacks affecting the brainstem are more common in pediatric MS [33].
- Recovery after a clinical exacerbation is shorter in younger patients compared to older children and adults, and tends to be complete after the initial attack [7, 10].
- A higher annualized relapse rate occurs in pediatric MS as compared to adult-onset disease.
- Relapses are frequent, but most children completely or near-completely recover from their first clinical attack. However, they also reach permanent disability at an earlier age [1, 12]
- Although disease progression is slower in pediatric MS and take longer to reach secondary progression, significant disability is accrued at a younger age [2, 23, 25, 26, 34, 35]
- Prognosis depends on severity and location of the attacks, and timing and frequency of relapses.
- The goal of therapy is to prevent relapses and ultimately disability.

References

[1] Waldman, A; Ness, J; Pohl, D; Simone, I; Anlar, B; Amato, M; et al. Pediatric multiple sclerosis: Clinical features and outcome. *Neurology*., 2016 Aug 30, 87(9 Suppl 2), S74-S81.

[2] Renoux, C; Vukusic, S; Mikaeloff, Y; Edan, G; Clanet, M; Dubois, B; et al. Natural History of Multiple Sclerosis with Childhood Onset. *NEJM*, 2007, 356(25), 2603-13.

[3] Ferreira, M; Machado, M; Dantas, M; Moreira, Á; Souza, A. Pediatric multiple sclerosis: analysis of clinical and epidemiological aspects according to National MS Society Consensus 2007. *Arquivos de Neuro-Psiquiatria*, 2008, 66(3b), 665-70.

[4] Belman, A; Krupp, L; Olsen, C; Rose, J; Aaen, G; Benson, L; et al. Characteristics of Children and Adolescents With Multiple Sclerosis. *Pediatrics.*, 2016 Jul, 138(1), pii, e20160120.

[5] Fenichel, G. *Clinical pediatric neurology*, 1st ed. Philadelphia, PA: Saunders Elsevier, 2009.

[6] Sindern, E; Haas, J; Stark, E; Wurster, U. Early onset MS under the age of 16: clinical and paraclinical features. *Acta Neurol Scand*, 1992, 86, 280–4.

[7] Ruggieri, M; Polizzi, A; Pavone, L; Grimaldi, LME. Multiple sclerosis in children under 6 years of age. *Neurology*, 1999, 53, 478-84.

[8] Gusev, E; Boiko, A; Bikova, O; Maslova, O; Guseva, M; Boiko, S; et al. The natural history of early onset multiple sclerosis: comparison of data from Moscow and Vancouver. *Clinical Neurology and Neurosurgery*, 2002, 104(3), 203-7.

[9] Chitnis, T; Glanz, B; Jaffin, S; Healy, B. Demographics of pediatric-onset multiple sclerosis in an MS center population from the Northeastern United States. *Multiple Sclerosis Journal*, 2009, 15(5), 627-31.

[10] Duquette, P; Murray, TJ; Pleines, I; et al. Multiple sclerosis in childhood: clinical profile in 125 patients. *J Pediatr*, 1987, 111, 359-33.

[11] Hanefeld, F; Bauer, H; Christen, H; Kruse, B; Bruhn, H; Frahm, J. Multiple sclerosis in childhood: Report of 15 cases. *Brain and Development*, 1991, 13(6), 410-6.

[12] Boiko, A; Vorobeychik, G; Paty, D; Devonshire, V; Sadovnick, D. the UBC MS Clinic Neurologists. Early onset multiple sclerosis: A longitudinal study. *Neurology*, 2002, 59(7), 1006-10.

[13] Benson, L; Healy, B; Gorman, M; Baruch, N; Gholipour, T; Musallam, A; et al. Elevated relapse rates in pediatric compared to adult MS persist for at least 6 years. *Multiple Sclerosis and Related Disorders*, 2014, 3(2), 186-93.

[14] Fragoso, Y; Ferreira, M; Morales, N; Arruda, W; Brooks, J; Carneiro, D; et al. Multiple sclerosis starting before the age of 18 years: the Brazilian experience. *Arquivos de Neuro-Psiquiatria*, 2013, 71(10), 783-7.

[15] Banwell, B; Ghezzi, A; Bar-Or, A; Mikaeloff, Y; Tardieu, M. Multiple sclerosis in children: clinical diagnosis, therapeutic strategies, and future directions. *The Lancet Neurology*, 2007, 6(10), 887-902.

[16] Amato, M; Krupp, L; Charvet, L; Penner, I; Till, C. Pediatric multiple sclerosis. *Neurology*, 2016, 87(9 Supplement 2), S82-S87.

[17] Krysko, K; O'Connor, P. Quality of Life, Cognition and Mood in Adults with Pediatric Multiple Sclerosis. *Canadian Journal of Neurological Sciences/Journal Canadien des Sciences Neurologiques*, 2016, 43(03), 368-74.

[18] Chitnis, T; Ghezzi, A; Bajer-Kornek, B; Boyko, A; Giovannoni, G; Pohl, D. Pediatric multiple sclerosis: Escalation and emerging treatments. *Neurology*, 2016, 87(9 Supplement 2), S103-S109.

[19] https://www.msif.org/wp-content/uploads/2016/08/Pediatric-MS-and-other-demyelinating-disorders-in-childhood-English.pdf. MS International federation webpage. Last accessed, June 3rd 2017.

[20] Suppiej, A; Cainelli, E. Cognitive dysfunction in pediatric multiple sclerosis. *Neuropsychiatric Disease and Treatment*, 2014, 10, 1385-92.

[21] Yeh, E; Chitnis, T; Krupp, L; Ness, J; Chabas, D; Kuntz, N et al. Pediatric multiple sclerosis. *Nature Reviews Neurology*, 2009, 5(11), 621-31.

[22] Hintzen, R; Dale, R; Neuteboom, R; Mar, S; Banwell, B. Pediatric acquired CNS demyelinating syndromes. Features associated with multiple sclerosis. *Neurology*, 2016, 87(9 Supplement 2), S67-S73.

[23] Ozakbas, S; Idiman, E; Baklan, B; Yulug, B. Childhood and juvenile onset multiple sclerosis: clinical and paraclinical features. *Brain and Development*, 2003, 25(4), 233-6.

[24] Huppke, B; Ellenberger, D; Rosewich, H; Friede, T; Gärtner, J; Huppke, P. Clinical presentation of pediatric multiple sclerosis before puberty. *European Journal of Neurology*, 2013, 21(3), 441-6.

[25] Gorman, M; Healy, B; Polgar-Turcsanyi, M; Chitnis, T. Increased Relapse Rate in Pediatric-Onset Compared With Adult-Onset Multiple Sclerosis. *Archives of Neurology*, 2009, 66(1).

[26] Simone, I; Carrara, D; Tortorella, C; Liguori, M; Lepore, V; Pellegrini, F; et al. Course and prognosis in early-onset MS, Comparison with adult-onset forms. *Neurology*, 2002, 59(12), 1922-8.

[27] Pena, J; Lotze, T. Pediatric Multiple Sclerosis: Current Concepts and Consensus Definitions. *Autoimmune Diseases*, 2013, 2013, 1-12.

[28] Wilejto, M; Shroff, M; Buncic, J; Kennedy, J; Goia, C; Banwell, B. The clinical features, MRI findings, and outcome of optic neuritis in children. *Neurology*, 2006, 67(2), 258-62.

[29] Lucchinetti, C; Kiers, L; O'Duffy, A; Gomez, M; Cross, S; Leavitt, J; et al. Risk factors for developing multiple sclerosis after childhood optic neuritis. *Neurology*, 1997, 49(5), 1413-8.

[30] Alroughani, R; Ahmed, S; Al-Hashel, J. Pediatric-Onset Multiple Sclerosis Disease Progression in Kuwait: A Retrospective Analysis. *Pediatric Neurology*, 2015, 53(6), 508-12.

[31] Mikaeloff, Y; Suissa, S; Vallée, L; Lubetzki, C; Ponsot, G; Confavreux, C; et al. First episode of acute CNS inflammatory demyelination in childhood: prognostic factors for multiple sclerosis and disability. *The Journal of Pediatrics*, 2004, 144(2), 246-52.

[32] Derle, E; Kurne, A; Konuşkan, B; Karabudak, R; Anlar, B. Unfavorable outcome of pediatric onset multiple sclerosis: Follow-up in the pediatric and adult neurology departments of one referral

center, in Turkey. *Multiple Sclerosis and Related Disorders*, 2016, 9, 1-4.

[33] Ghezzi, A; Deplano, V; Faroni, J; et al. Multiple sclerosis in childhood: clinical features of 149 cases. *Mult Scler*, 1997, 3, 43-6.

[34] El-Salem, K; Khader, Y. Comparison of the natural history and prognostic features of early onset and adult onset multiple sclerosis in Jordanian population. *Clinical Neurology and Neurosurgery*, 2007, 109(1), 32-7.

[35] Pinhas-Hamiel, O; Barak, Y; Siev-Ner, I; Achiron, A. Juvenile multiple sclerosis, Clinical features and prognostic characteristics. *The Journal of Pediatrics*, 1998, 132(4), 735-7.

In: Multiple Sclerosis in Children … ISBN: 978-1-53612-979-3
Editors: H. Omar and J. Chalkley

Chapter 4

TREATMENT OF PEDIATRIC MULTIPLE SCLEROSIS

Joshua Chalkley, DO
Department of Neurology Neuroimmunology/
Multiple Sclerosis Division, University of Kentucky,
Lexington, Kentucky, US

ABSTRACT

The treatment of multiple sclerosis has undergone a major revolution over the last decade. In many patients, clinicians are able to keep the disease under control, however the literature in pediatric disease has lagged behind its adult counterparts. The purpose of this paper is to review the literature on the treatment of pediatric multiple sclerosis and to discuss developing treatment approaches in dealing with the pediatric population.

Keywords: pediatric multiple sclerosis, treatment of pediatric multiple sclerosis, disease modifying therapy

INTRODUCTION

The last two decades have seen a revolution in the treatment of multiple sclerosis. The number of disease modifying therapies and subsequent complexity of treatment options bring new hope to those living with multiple sclerosis, and the providers caring for them. However, despite the significant improvement of available treatment options most of these drugs have not been studied in the pediatric population. There is little controlled trial data examining treatment efficacy in children. Treatment implications in the pediatric population could be potentially far reaching given their continued physical and neurologic development. Interferons, glatiramer acetate, fingolimod, teriflunimide, dimethyl fumarate, natalizumab, daclizumab, alemtuzumab, and ocrelizumab are currently FDA approved for multiple sclerosis. There is also good trial data for cyclophosphamide, and rituximab with these drugs being used off label for multiple sclerosis [1, 2]. However, despite our range of treatment options in the adult population pediatric studies have been lagging. Rigorous placebo-controlled trials are for the most part absent in the pediatric literature. However, there is treatment data for a number of agents with larger prospective studies underway.

Despite increasing treatment options there are still significant gaps in the treatment of multiple sclerosis. As the treatment of MS improved the concept of a disease free state or no evidence of disease activity has emerged. No evidence of disease activity or NEDA is defined as no clinical relapse, no new symptoms, no progression of disability, and no MRI activity. One study looking at 7-year treatment data using the CLIMB database showed only 7.9% met these criteria at the end of seven years [3]. NEDA has not been systematically studied in pediatric populations. Although there is been increasing success in the treatment of the inflammatory component of multiple sclerosis, progressive disease remains a treatment conundrum. There are drugs showing promise in the treatment of progressive disease (Rituximab, ocrelizumab, biotin, etc.) for many this remains a devastating aspect of disease. To date we have no drugs which can repair the nervous system. There are also significant gaps and treatment knowledge on when we should stop therapy and in predicting who would have more aggressive disease versus a more benign course. The focus on pediatric disease in general and more specifically pediatric multiple sclerosis is risen to the forefront in the recent years. Pediatric multiple sclerosis was initially thought to be exceedingly rare but numerous studies have shown this may more common than initially thought. Several large database studies and shown the incidence of pediatric MS to be higher than predicted [4-6]. In the United States there was a large California database that was reported as showing incidence of pediatric MS hip 0.51/100,000[6]. In Canada the incidence is 1.8/1000,000 and in Germany estimated incidence of pediatric MS is 0.3/100,000 [7]. For the most part pediatric multiple sclerosis is adolescent disease with the most common major diagnosis around the age of 15. Prepubertal multiple sclerosis remains very rare with the age of two being the youngest case to date [2].

Pediatric multiple sclerosis appears to be more inflammatory than seen in adult populations. In retrospective studies analyzed annualized relapse rate of pediatric onset MS is between 0.38 and 0.87 [8, 5]. Another study looking Pediatric patients with multiple sclerosis at an academic Medical Center MS found a 2-3 fold higher relapse rate during her first 3 years disease than they're adult counterparts [9]. Despite her higher frequency of relapse, the overall improvement appears to be more rapid than what seen in adult populations. The disability progression varies from individual to individual and pediatric patients appear to have lower disability score was then compared to the adult counterparts with the same duration of disease [10, 5]. Although it appears that children with multiple sclerosis take longer to develop disability given early onset of disease they typically will reach higher EDSS scores approximately 10 years younger than they're adult counterparts. This can be especially problematic given these young adults would typically be moving into the most productive adult years. The impact of using disease modifying therapies in pediatric present patients has not been studied in the longitudinal way.

Cognitive dysfunction is one of the most common features of pediatric multiple sclerosis [11-13]. One study of 37 children with multiple sclerosis showed 60% these children had cognitive difficulties in one major domain and 35% had cognitive difficulties in two major domains [12]. Cognitive deficits are especially important in pediatric patients giving her ongoing developing brain as well as there is patients continued education. The areas are most commonly affected more complex attention, delayed recall, visual memory, and naming. Most children have relatively intact verbal fluency and immediate recall [13, 14].

In summary pediatric patients tend to have a more aggressive onset at the beginning of their disease with significant inflammation. They tend to have more relapses than their adult counterparts as well as more active MRI findings. Given the highly inflammatory nature of the disease in conjunction with a lifelong illness treatment needs to be initiated in a timely manner. Today most effective treatments are targeted to treat inflammation, which may be especially important pediatric patients.

The treatment of pediatric multiple sclerosis is divided into 2 major categories. The first is to treat acute inflammation during an attack. The second, is to prevent future attacks through the advance of disease modifying therapy. Disease modifying therapy (DMT) is become the mainstay of the treatment of multiple sclerosis in the hopes of preventing future attacks, progression of disability and overall improved quality of life. All of the disease modifying therapies to date target a specific part of the immune system in hopes of decreasing the inflammatory aspects of multiple sclerosis. DMT has revolutionized treatment of multiple sclerosis and a certain percentage of the population is able to prevent disease progression. Although these medications have improved the treatment of multiple sclerosis there is still significant limitations. The medications are complex and require rigorous specialize monitoring and several of the drugs can have severe potentially life-threatening side effects. A significant percentage of the population do not respond to these medications. This is especially true in pediatric populations were as much as 30%-45% of these patients will need to be switched on to a stronger agent for disease progression or side effects [15]. Disease modifying therapies have been studied extensively in the adult populations, but there is less literature in pediatrics. There is a consensus in the pediatric population to treat with first line therapies including glatiramer acetate and interferons first. If the patient has intolerance or failure of these first-line drugs, then he can consider second line treatments.

SELECTION OF AGENTS

Given the increased complexity and options in the treatment of multiple sclerosis the selection of disease modifying therapy has become increasingly complicated. Traditionally in academic literature the terminology of first versus second line therapy has dominated. However, the concept of induction versus escalation therapy is currently replacing this model. Escalation therapy is the stepwise progression of less potent agents to more aggressive treatment strategies. Typically, this is starting with either interferon or glatiramer acetate and if the patient fails these medications to then move to a more potent drug. Induction therapy is the opposite approach starting with a potent agent followed possibly by de-escalation after stabilization. Currently there is insignificant data to support one approach over the other. There is little in the way of validated outcome predictors in patients with multiple sclerosis. There is essentially no data in pediatric literature in regards to outcome predictors.

The field in general is moving towards a more personalized approach one selecting disease modifying therapy. This personalized approach takes into account the individuals overall picture of disease, their personal preferences and their treatment goals in regards to their disease.

given chemical similarity to rituximab this may be a promising medication for the pediatric population. In the adult clinical trials that showed significant reduction in relapse rates as well as disability progression and MRI findings. Ocrelizumab will also be approved for progressive forms of multiple sclerosis [53]. Ocrelizumab had a good safety profile in adult populations with some infusion related reactions. There is likely a small risk of increased infection, but these tended to be mild in the adult trials. To date there were no cases of PML associated with ocrelizumab, but given is chemical similarity of rituximab there is likely a small risk of PML [53].

Alemtuzumab

Alemtuzumab is reserved for aggressive forms multiple sclerosis in adult populations. It is a monoclonal antibody targeting CD52 B cells. It was effective in decreasing relapse rates, decreasing MRI activity and disability progression in adult populations but is never been studied in the pediatric population. Given its potentially serious side effect profile it's reserved for patients who have failed at least 2 forms of other disease modifying therapies [54]. The incidence of infusion related reactions is significant including potentially severe anaphylactic shock. Approximately a third of patients will develop other autoimmune disease related to the use of this medication. Most of his was thyroid disease which is relatively easily treated there have been cases of fatal ITP as well as autoimmune kidney disease. These this medication requires close monitoring for long periods of time. All effective given its potential toxicity is reserved for refractory disease. There is no data available for treatment in pediatric populations [54].

Mitoxantrone

Mitoxantrone is a synthetic anthracenedione which has multiple effects on the immune system. It suppresses the proliferation of T cells, B cells,

Table 1. FDA Approved Medications for Multiple Sclerosis

Medication	FDA Approval	Mechanism of Action	Dosing	Most Common Side Effects
Interferon beta	Treatment of relapsing forms of MS,	Regulate T cell response, decrease antigen presentation and T cell proliferation	Varying dosage and duration of dosing all injectable	Flu like symptoms, headaches, fatigue, injection site pain
Glatiramer acetate	Treatment of Relapsing forms of MS	Regulates T cell response, mimics myelin	20mg daily or 40mg three times weekly, by injection	Injection site pain, lipodystrophy
Teriflunomide	Treatment of relapsing forms of MS	Inhibits pyrimidine de nova synthesis which inhibits rapidly dividing cells including T cells, blocks transcription factors	7mg or 14mg oral daily	Headache, hair thinning, diarrhea, hepatic injury, tertogenic
Fingolimod	Relapsing forms of Ms	Sphigosine-1 receptor modulator, traps developing immune cells in peripheral lymph tissue	0.5mg oral daily	Bradycardia, elevated liver enzymes, macular edema, rare serious infections including PML,
Dimethyl fumarate	Relapsing forms of MS	Rapidly attacked by glutathione, multiple possible actions including up regulating anti-inflammatory stress protein	240mg oral daily	Flushing, GI upset, lymphopenia, hepatic injury, rare cases of PML
daclizumab	Relapsing forms of MS	Humanized IgG1 MAD against IL-R chain	120mg once a month by injection	URI, rash, flu like symptoms, depression, hepatic injury, immune related conditions
natalizumab	Relapsing forms of MS	Works by adhesion to alpha4-integrin receptor blocking T cell migration into the CNS	300mg IV every month	PML
ocrelizumab	Primary progressive MS, Relapsing forms of MS	Anti CD20	600mg IV every 6 months, first dose given in 300mg two weeks apart	URI, UTI, possible increase in malignancy, possible increase risk of breast cancer,

Medication	FDA Approval	Mechanism of Action	Dosing	Most Common Side Effects
alemtuzumab	Relapsing forms of MS	Binds to CD52 B cells	12mg IV daily for five days, followed by 12mg per day for three days one year later	Infusion related reactions, secondary autoimmune disease ITP, immune related kidney disease, increased risk of malignancy, thyroid disease
mitoxantrone	Secondary progressive, progressive relapsing, worsening relapsing MS	Suppresses the proliferation of T cells, B cells and macrophages, impairs antigen presentation	12mg/m squared every three months max lifetime dose 140 mg/m squared	Nausea, hair loss, URI, UTI, cardiac damage, AML

Acute Treatment of Disease

Relapses are typically treated with IV methyl prednisolone 20/30 milligrams per kilogram with a maximum dose of 1 g daily. Treatment duration is typically 3-5 days followed occasionally by an oral prednisone taper. Adult data does not appear to support the need for corticosteroid taper after the completion of pulse corticosteroids. Occasionally with severe attacks or in incomplete response to steroids intravenous immunoglobulin 0.4 g/kg per day for 5 days her plasmapheresis can be considered. This may be reserved for severe attacks especially cervical cord involvement.

Disease Modifying Therapy

Interferon Beta

Beta interferons are commonly uses first-line treatments in pediatric MS. The exact mechanism of action is still poorly understood. These drugs probably work by combination of inhibiting pro-inflammatory cytokines, reduction of lymphocyte migration, in addition of down regulating reactive T cells, and possibly the promotion of anti-inflammatory mediators. These drugs have been rigorously studied in adult populations with an approximately 30% reduction relapse rate across trials [16-18].

There are no placebo-controlled prospective studies in pediatric multiple sclerosis. There are several retrospective case series which children was significant difference in sample size. These retrospective studies show similar reduction in relapse rate when compared to adult trials. Interferon is relatively well tolerated and safe in pediatric populations [19, 20]. Approximately 35-65% of patients will develop some flulike symptoms at the initiation of treatment. Besides the flulike symptoms there were also leukopenia, thrombocytopenia, anemia and elevation of liver enzymes. Injection site reactions and rarely injection site necrosis were reported. Depression is a well-known adult phenomenon related to interferon use but this is being poorly studied in pediatric populations. One retrospective study of subcutaneous interferon beta-1a was found have rates the depression proximally 2-4% [21, 22]. It appears that younger pediatric patients may be more susceptible to hepatic side effects than older children [19-22]. One retrospective study of interferon beta -1b found the children younger than age 10 had a 63% incidence of liver function test elevation was compared to their older counterparts only 10% had elevation of liver enzymes. Despite the difference in hepatic function flulike symptoms and injection site reactions were similar in both groups. The symptoms consistently showed a reduction relapse rate among patients treated with intramuscular beta interferon.

Dosing considerations are complicated in pediatric multiple sclerosis. There is no uniform dosing schedule and drug titration were not standardized. Most children studied were escalated to full dose although dosing was different throughout the trials. Neutralizing antibodies are a well-known phenomenon in adult patient's but there is data on the risk of pediatric patients developing neutralizing antibodies. There is one study suggesting that neutralizing antibodies in pediatric population are less common that in adult population.

Glatiramer Acetate

Glatiramer acetate is an acetate salt a mixture of sympathetic polypeptide seen in myelin basic protein. Glatiramer acetate is a complicated structure and likely works by the mimic of human myelin basic protein. It is suggested to induce a myelin specific response of suppressor T lymphocytes, inhibiting specific effector T lymphocytes and their action upon antigen presentation cells [23]. Glatiramer acetate has been used in adult MS populations for the better part of 2 decades. It is considered the safest disease modifying therapy with no significant side effects and no long-term blood monitoring. In adult populations is been compared to interferon and they're found to be equivocal in terms of disease modification [24]. There are several small studies looking at glatiramer acetate and safety. There were no major side effects and these groups although one patient had a transient systemic reaction and several patients had post injection site reactions [25]. There were no major side effects reported in these studies [26].

Natalizumab

Natalizumab is a humanized monoclonal antibody targeting alpha 4 integrin and approved for refractory MS in the adult population. Natalizumab blocs the migration of T and B cells into the central nervous system. In adults, studies natalizumab shows a robust anti-inflammatory effect [27]. There have been several small retrospective studies in pediatric populations [28-31]. One study done by Korenek and colleagues evaluated 20 children with highly active relapsing multiple sclerosis. There was reduction and analyze relapse rates, in EDSS scores, and the number of T2 lesions. 46% of these patients remained free of clinical disease with no MRI detectable disease during treatment. 37% of patients remained free of disease activity 2 years after the study [28]. There is another small study conducted by Ghezzi and colleagues who actively followed 19 pediatric patients with multiple sclerosis receiving natalizumab. Their annualized relapse rates decreased significantly although 30% continuing to experience attacks and there was evidence of MRI detectable disease in 7 of the 13 patients. These patients were slightly younger with an average age of 14.6 years as opposed to 16.7 years in the Korenek study. Given the higher rate of relapse in pediatric onset versus adult onset multiple sclerosis irrespective of the use of disease modifying therapy natalizumab was effective [31].

Adverse events with natalizumab treated patients were slightly higher than adults with is much is 15% of patients having some side effect in one study. There are several infections of the respiratory and urinary tracks that required antibiotic treatment however both of these infections minor. There was one patient who developed severe facial phlegmon. There was one patient who developed orchitis. There was some debate whether these infections were secondary to natalizumab [28].

These studies have significant limitations. Some of the limitations of the study include a retrospective design, with clinical and laboratory and radiologic evaluations at nonuniform times. They use nonuniform protocols small number patient's studied. Most of the patients studied were above the age of 12 and there is very limited data on prepubertal patient's with natalizumab.

The use of natalizumab is limited by the risk of progressive multifocal leukoencephalopathy (PML). There is a risk stratification protocol developed for adult patients. The risk of PML increases with prior immunosuppressant use, duration of treatment greater than 24 months, and the presence of anti-JCV virus titer antibodies [32]. Natalizumab is relatively safe in JCV negative individuals. There is some recent data that overall risk of PML may have been initially underestimated. Berger and Fox reviewed the risk stratification for natalizumab in 2016 and found if patient's had duration of treatment greater than 24 months, prior immunosuppressant therapy, and they were JC virus positive the risk of developing PML was approximately 1 in 44 [33]. There were no cases of PML in pediatric treated populations but these numbers are very small. Given MS is a lifelong disease close monitoring of JC virus titers are needed in pediatric populations.

Two large population based studies demonstrated that adolescence have lower rates of JC virus infection than adults [34, 35]. Despite this the specifics of JC virus infection rates of pediatric patients with MS our unknown. Natalizumab appears to be effective in the pediatric population, however should likely be reserved for highly active disease. [28-31].

Daclizumab

Daclizumab is a humanized monoclonal antibody specific for interleukin-2 (IL)-2 receptor alpha chain. It is FDA approved for the treatment of refractory MS in adults. Daclizumab blocks the interleukin-2 binding site on the interleukin-2R alpha chain. Daclizumab is effective in the treatment of relapse remitting multiple sclerosis in adults [36]. In one small study 7 children with aggressive multiple sclerosis with breakthrough disease on standard platform agents were given Daclizumab. The treatment group was largely in combination with interferon beta 1A although two patients were treated with daclizumab monotherapy. Treated patient showed overall reductions in analyze relapse rates and all patient's improvement on the expanded disability status scale scores. Overall daclizumab was well tolerated with no serious side effects [37].

There are limitations to this case series this was an open label treatment series. These patients were evaluated clinically and radiographically in nonuniform times using nonuniform MRI protocols, which is reflective of clinical practice. Only 2 of these patients used daclizumab alone, and were most treated in combination with interferon. Despite the limitations of this study it does provide treatment data in patients with aggressive MS. Daclizumab May be an important add-on agent as well as affective and monotherapy for patients with treatment refractory multiple sclerosis [37].

Although there are other second line treatment options to daclizumab is an attractive option in pediatric patients. Compared with chemotherapy daclizumab is not known to cause infertility or secondary malignancies both of which are increased concern in pediatric populations. Progressive multifocal leukoencephalopathy has not been reported in daclizumab. Both natalizumab and rituximab have been associated with PML. In addition, daclizumab has been used safely in pediatric patients with solid organ transplantation. There are ongoing concerns mostly from the adult literature with elevated liver enzymes, psoriasis, infections, and rash that would require extended close monitoring. As with the use of all monoclonal's there is concern about the long-term consequences of these drugs which is especially pertinent in pediatric populations.

Rituximab

Rituximab is a monoclonal antibody targeting CD 20 receptors and activated B cells. Rituximab is not FDA approved for treatment of multiple sclerosis, but is used off label in adult populations, and there is good data showing efficacy in adult populations [38]. Recently, Ocrelizumab which is a monoclonal antibody with similar structure and mechanism of action as rituximab was FDA approved for multiple sclerosis this year. Both of these drugs have shown to decrease relapse rates as well as decrease in active MRI lesions in adult populations [38, 39]. There is significant data on rituximab for lymphoma rheumatoid arthritis and other immune related conditions. There are no placebo-controlled trials in pediatric populations.

There are case series in pediatric patients with rituximab as well as for other central nervous system inflammatory diseases. These studies have shown rituximab to be effective and overall well tolerated. None of these patients had a relapse with a median treatment duration of 23.6 months. Another small retrospective study with rituximab with 11 pediatric patients, 8 patients with neuromyelitis optica and 3 patients with MS, two of the three children with multiple sclerosis remained relapse free at follow-up although one patient continued to have relapses. In this small trial in both the patient's with neuromyelitis optica and multiple sclerosis the treatment was well tolerated with no serious side effects. There were no serious infections reported in these small studies [40-42]. Overall rituximab has a good safety profile in both adult children. There is slight increased risk of infection although for the most part these are minor. There have been cases of PML associated with rituximab in a patient with lups but there are no cases to date of PML with rituximab in multiple sclerosis populations, although this risk likely exists [43]. There are cases of PML in association with others disease which is further muddied by the fact the patients were often on multiple immunosuppressant agents including prednisone, methotrexate and other immune related medications [44]. The risk and pediatric populations is probably small there is very limited data in this subject. There is some concern given rituximab has long-lasting effects on the immune system that these results may last for many years.

Cyclophosphamide

Cyclophosphamide is alkylating chemotherapeutic agent binds to DNA and interferes with mitosis, and cell replication. Cyclophosphamide decreases pro-inflammatory T helper cell, and cytokines, causes the secretion of anti-inflammatory Th2 cytokines IL-4 and IL-10 in both CSF blood. Cyclophosphamide was the first drug to show a possible disease modifying affect in multiple sclerosis after Hauser, Weiner and colleges used pulse dose cyclophosphamide in the treatment of MS in 1983 [45, 46]. There is retrospective data looking at pulse dose or induction therapy cyclophosphamide in pediatric literature. In the majority of cases there was decrease relapse frequency as well as EDSS improvement one year for initiation of cyclophosphamide therapy [47]. In adult literature it appears that patients under the age of 40 were better responders to nose or age of 40 wakening some credence this may be a more potent anti-inflammatory drug. This may be evidence importance given children have a more aggressive inflammatory component in the disease.

Despite cyclophosphamide efficacy does have significant risks as well as a difficult side effect profile. In retrospective pediatric literature cyclophosphamide was associated with vomiting, transient alopecia, osteoporosis, and amenorrhea. One patient developed bladder carcinoma that was successfully treated. Hemorrhagic cystitis and bladder carcinoma overall known side effects of cyclophosphamide therapy [47]. Another benefit of cyclophosphamide therapy as there is significant experience in the pediatric literature with other immune related diseases as well as pediatric leukemia which can help in for management of children with multiple sclerosis. Given cyclophosphamide's more frequent use in other pediatric diseases this may give some guidance in regards to dosing and potential side effects. Patient's on cyclophosphamide therapy need to be monitored for the risk of severe adverse events including amenorrhea, infections, stability, hemorrhagic cystitis, bladder cancer, and other malignancies. Given his overall toxicity cyclophosphamide is not an appropriate first line therapy that may be useful as a salvage therapy and children who are experiencing increasing disability secondary to their disease.

Fingolimod

Fingolimod is a sphingosine-1-phosphate receptor modulator which works by trapping developing lymphocytes and peripheral lymph tissue. Fingolimod is a once a day oral medication, and showed reduction relapse rate, MRI activity and disability progression and adults [48]. Fingolimod showed significant efficacy in the adult population there is very little data in regards to pediatric MS. Fingolimod is generally well tolerated but can cause bradycardia in a small percentage of patients. It has also been associated with macular edema as well as rare opportunistic infections and malignancies. There've been cases of Kaposi sarcoma and 9 total cases of progressive multifocal leukoencephalopathy to date.

There is some literature available in the use of fingolimod in pediatric populations. One retrospective study followed 17 children with aggressive MS. These patients all had active disease. In this study there was a reduction in relapse rate as well as MRI activity. Overall these small studies have shown efficacy as well as good safety data although the total numbers are small [48, 49].

Although to date most of the literature has been retrospective the PARADIGMS study will be the first double blinded active controlled trial in pediatric MS. The study hopes to recruit 190 pediatric patients ranging from age 10-18 and will be placed on either interferon or fingolimod. This will be the first prospective randomized controlled study in pediatric multiple sclerosis. [49].

Dimethyl Fumarate

Dimethyl fumarate has a poorly understood mechanism of action. It is thought to work by decreasing cytokine production, and prevents lymphocyte migration through the blood brain barrier. This is a twice a day oral medication which is shown to be ineffective in adult populations. In terms of side effects, it is most commonly associated with nausea, and flushing. These effects may be diminished by taking the medication with fatty foods. In terms of serious side effects occasionally can cause lymphopenia as well as hepatic injury. There've been several cases of progressive multifocal leukoencephalopathy in both dimethyl fumarate and in other fumaric acid formulations used in Europe for psoriatic arthritis [50].

There is some limited data using dimethyl fumarate in pediatric populations. One retrospective study by Makhani and colleagues followed 13 children on dimethyl fumarate. In five of the children this was first line therapy. 89% had decreased or stabilized relapse rates as well as no disability progression. New T2 lesions were seen in three of the children [51]. The most common side effects were nausea, facial flushing, and fatigue which is consistent with the adult population. There was no lymphopenia or elevation in liver enzymes in this small retrospective study [51]. This study has limitations given it retrospective design, small size, non-uniform dosing, and that not all children were imaged, but dimethyl fumarate does appear to be safe and effective in pediatric populations. There is ongoing placebo controlled trials evaluating the efficacy of dimethyl fumarate in pediatric populations [49].

Teriflunomide

Teriflunomide, is a pyrimidine synthesis inhibitor used in the treatment of multiple sclerosis. Teriflunomide Inhibits pyrimidine de nova synthesis which consequently inhibits rapidly dividing cells including T cells. It also blocks transcription factors including NF-kB. To date there's been no studies with children but it was shown to be effective in adult multiple sclerosis. For the most part this drug is relatively well-tolerated although can cause some GI upset as well as alopecia. In terms of serious side effects, it's been associated with hepatic toxicity requiring frequent blood monitoring for the first six months and every six months thereafter. This may be particularly difficult in teenage populations especially in reproductive age women given this is a category X for pregnancy. This drug is also past and seminal fluid and has an unknown teratogenic, possibly even in the male population [52].

There is limited data on its use in children but there is one phase 3 trial underway now. The TERIKIDS trial is a 2 year randomized, double blinded placebo controlled, parallel group trial examining the effectiveness in teriflunomide in children with MS ages 10-17. This multicenter trial will hopefully provide important additional information on the treatment of pediatric MS with teriflunomide [49].

Ocrelizumab

Ocrelizumab is a humanized monoclonal antibody similar to rituximab targeting CD20 B cells. There are clinical trials ongoing to monitor its effect in children. The adult studies show robust therapeutic effect and

and macrophages. Mitoxantrone impairs antigen presentation and decreases macrophage mediated myelin degradation. Mitoxantrone is FDA approved for adults with aggressive relapsing forms of MS and secondary progressive MS. There is some data for its use in pediatric patients. Etamadifar and collogues gave mitoxantrone to 19 children with aggressive MS. After a median follow up period of 30 months, 74% were relapse free, and 84% and improvement in EDSS. Adverse events included nausea and vomiting, alopecia, palpitation, fatigue cardiomyopathy and mild leukopenia. All adverse events were mild and transient [55].

Mitoxantrone is rarely used given its overall toxicity, however it may be a useful medication in severe refractory MS. Another advantage of mitoxantrone is its broad effect on the immune system. However, serious thought needs to be given to its use given its increased risk of malignancy as well as cardiotoxicity which limit its overall usefulness in multiple sclerosis. Given the myriad of other treatment options mitoxantrone is rarely used [55].

Symptomatic Management

Multiple sclerosis is a lifelong disease that requires multidisciplinary approach to fully address the needs of these patients. Patients with multiple sclerosis of a several wife variety of symptoms including chronic pain, cognitive dysfunction, depression, fatigue, urinary urgency, urinary hesitancy, pain, spasticity, and a wide variety of neurologic complaints. Symptomatic management and rehabilitation will be covered and later chapters of this book, but is important to briefly mention in multidisciplinary approach is probably the best avenue to deal with agents with complex disease states. This may be especially true in pediatric populations when patients who often need access to specialty care. Multiple subspecialists or needed including physical medicine and rehabilitation, pain medicine, neuro-ophthalmology, neurology, psychiatry, psychology, theatrics and social work.

MOVING FORWARD

Despite the paucity of clinical trial literature and pediatric multiple sclerosis there's been recent mandates in both United States in Europe requiring pediatric studies and new biological agents. Hopefully these new mandates will lead to expanding treatment data in pediatric populations. There are significant challenges in conducting clinical trials in pediatric populations given their small numbers, poorly understood disease state, and ethical impractical concerns related to treatment of pediatric populations.

The international pediatric clinical trials Summit from the staring committee of the international pediatric MS study group met in 2012 which included multiple academic experts in the field pediatric MS as well as the FDA and European medicine agencies. Based on the findings of this meeting they recommended studies with outcome measures to include clinical, cognitive an MRI data to be reviewed in pediatric MS clinic will trials this at those important for the development of international unified long-term drug registry. Hopefully this will spur an increasing clinical trial data focused on children with multiple sclerosis [49].

The international Pediatric Study Group recommended the exposure of novel MS drugs be in the context of carefully designed clinical trials, placebo controlled trials should be of brief duration with rigorous monitoring as well as rescue strategy for children with relapse. These studies should include development and growth parameters, as well as long-term impact on fertility. Contraceptive use and close pregnancy monitoring in appropriate populations. Some additional recommendations include randomized controlled trials are necessary from a drug approval standpoint. Studies should include children less than 10 years of age. Relapse should be clinically meaningful outcome measure. These studies should include a psychological battery that is sensitive to cognitive deficits in pediatric MS. There is need for a prospective registry to collect safety and clinical outcomes in patients exposed to therapies to evaluate long-term impact [56, 49].

Conclusion

Despite the absence of placebo-controlled trials in multiple sclerosis there is good data to support treatment of patients with pediatric multiple sclerosis. As when initiating any treatment, it is vital to weight the risks and benefits of the medication versus the long-term effects disease. Pediatric multiple sclerosis does not tend to be a benign entity patients have higher relapse rates than in the adult population and given the long duration of the disease treatment is appropriate. There is good data for the use of beta interferons, glatiramer acetate, daclizumab, daclizumab and interferon in combination, rituximab and natalizumab. Although these studies are small they do show a treatment effect in pediatric multiple sclerosis.

Currently interferons and glatiramer acetate are recommended as first-line treatments in pediatric populations. However, there is a growing concern this may be too conservative approach in highly inflammatory patients. It is clear from the literature that pediatric populations have a higher relapse rate than in adult populations. As many as 30% of patients do not tolerate first-line treatments either due to relapse or intolerance of the medications. If patient's fail first-line treatment with either interferon or glatiramer acetate there is good literature to support the use of rituximab, cyclophosphamide, natalizumab, daclizumab either as a single agent or in combination with interferon therapy and there is some limited data using fingolimod. With the new focus on pediatric inclusion in clinical trials there will be new data to better guide the clinician in the selection of agents over the next decade.

References

[1] Hauser, SL; Waubant, E; Arnold, DL. B-cell depletion with rituximab in relapsin-remitting multiple sclerosis. *N Engl J Med*, 2008, 358, 676-688.

[2] Makhani, N; Gorman, MP; Branson, HM; Stazzone, L; Banwell, BL; Chitnis, T. Cyclophosphamide therapi in pediartic multiple scleroiss. *Neurology*, 2009, 72, 2076-82.

[3] Rostein, DL; Healy, BC; Malik, MT; Chitnis, T; Weiner, HL. Evaluation of no evidence of disease activity 7-year longidutonal multiple sclerosis cohort. *JAMA Neurology*, 2015, 72, 152-8.

[4] Chitnis, T; Glanz, B; Jaffin, S; Healy, B. Demographics of pediatric onset multiple sclerosis in a na MS center populationg from the Northeastern United States. *Mult Scler*, 2009, 15, 627-31.

[5] Chitnis, T. Disease-Modifying therapy of pediatric multiple sclerosis. *Neurotherapuetics*, 2013, 10, 89-96.

[6] Langer-Gould, A; Zhang, JL; Chung, J; Yeung, Y; WAubant, E; Yao, J. Incidence of acquired CNS demyelinating syndromes in a multiethnic cohort of children. *Neurology*, 20111, 77, 1143-8.

[7] Banwell, B; Kennedy, J; Sadovnick, D. Incidence of acquired demylenation of the CNS in Canadian children. *Neurology*, 2009, 72, 232-9.

[8] Sindern, E; Haas, J; Stark, E; Wurster, U. Early onset MS under the age of 16: clinical and paraclinical features. *Acta Neurol Scand*, 1992, 86, 280-4.

[9] Gorman, MP; Healy, BC; Polgar-Turcsanyi, M; Chitnis, T. Increased relapse rate in pediatric-onset compared with adult-onset multiple sclerosis. *Arch Neurol*, 2009, 66, 54-9.

[10] Simone, IL; Carrara, D; Tortorella, C. Course and prognosis in early-onset MS: comparison with adult-onset forms. *Neurology*, 2002, 59, 1922-8.

[11] Banwell, BL; Anderson, PE. The cognitive burden of multiple sclerosis in children. *Neurology*, 2005, 64, 891-4.

[12] MacAllister, WS; Belman, AL; MIlazzo, M. Cognitive functioningi n children and adolescents with multiple sclerosis. *Neurology*, 2005, 64, 1422-5.

[13] Amato, MP; Goretti, B; Ghezzi, A. Cognitive and pychosocial features of childrood and juvenile MS. *Neurology*, 2008, 71, 1891-7.

[14] Amato, MP;Goretti, B. Ghezzzi. Cognitive and psychosocial features in chilhood and juvenile MS: two-yearfollo-up. *Neurology*, 2010, 75, 1134-40.

[15] Yeh, EA;Waubant, E; Krupp, LB. Multiple Sclerosis therapies in pediatric patient with refractory multiple sclerosis. *Arch Neurol*, 2010, 68, 437-44.

[16] Group IMSS. Interferon beta1b is effective in relapsing-remitting multiple sclerosis. I clinical results of a multicenter randomized double blind, placebo-controlled trial. *Neurology*, 1993, 655-61.

[17] Jacobs, L; Cookfair, D; Rudick, R. Intramuscular interferon beta1a for disease progression relapsing multiple sclerosis. *Ann Neurol*, 1996, 39, 285-94.

[18] Group PRISMS. Randomized, double-blind, placebo-controlled study of inteferon beta 1a in relapsing/remitting multiple sclerosis. *Lancet*, 1998, 352, 1498-1504.

[19] Mikaeloff, Y; Moreau, T; Bebouverie, M. Interferon-beta treatment in patients with childhood-onset multiple sclerosis. *J Pediatr*, 2001, 139, 443-6.

[20] Banwell, B; Reder, AT; Krupp, L. Safety and tolerability of interferon beta-1b in pediatric multiple sclerosis. *Neurology*, 2006, 66, 472-6.

[21] Pohl, D; Rostasy, K; Gartner, J; HAnefeld, F. Treament of early onset multiple sclerosis with subcutaneous interferon beta-1a. *Neurology*, 2005, 645, 888-890.

[22] Tenembaum, SN; Segura, JM. Interferon beta-1a treatmetnt in childhood and jevenile-onset multiple sclerosis. *Neurology*, 2006, 67, 511-3.

[23] Dhib-Jalbut, S. Sustained immunolgical effects of Glatiramer acetate in patients with multple sclerosis treated for over 6 years. *J Neurol Sci*, 2002, 201, 71-7.

[24] La Manita, L; Di Pietrantoni, C; Rovaris, M. Interferons-beta versus Glatiramer Acetate for relpase remitting multiple sclerosis. *Conchrane Database Syst Rev.*, 2016, Nov 24, 11.

[25] Kornek, B; Bernert, G; Balassy, C. Glatiramer acetate treatme in patints with childhoo and juvenile onset multple sclerosis. *Neuropediatrics*, 2003, 34, 120-6.

[26] Ghezzi, A; Amato, MP; Capobianco, M. Disease-modifying drugs in childhoo-juvenile multiple sclerosis: results of an Italian co-operative study. *Mult Scler*, 2005, 11, 420-4.

[27] Polman, CH; O'Conner, PW; Havrdova, E. A randomized, placebo-controlled trial of natalizumab for relapsing multiple sclerosis. *N Eng J Med*, 2006, 354, 899-910.

[28] Kornek, B; Aboul-Enein, F; Rostasy, K. Natalizumab therapy for highly active pediatric multiple sclerosis. *JAMA Neurol.*, 2013, 70, 469-75.

[29] Huppke, P; Stark, W; Zurcher, C. Natalizumab in children with multiple sclerosis. *Arch Neurol*, 2008, 65, 1655-8.

[30] Borriello, G; Prosperini, L; Luchetti, A; Pozzili, C. Natalizumab treatment in pediatric multiple sclerosis: acase report. *Eur J paediatr Neurol*, 2009, 13, 67-71.

[31] Ghezzi, A; Pozzili, C; Grimaldi, LM. Safety and efficacy of natalizumab in children with multiple sclerosis. *Neurology*, 2010, 75, 912-7.

[32] Gorelik, L; Lerner, M; Bexler, S. Anti-JC virus antibodies: implications for PML risk stratification. *Ann Neurol*, 2010, 68, 295-303.

[33] Berger, JR; Fox, R. Reassessing the risk of natalizumab associated PML. *J neurovirol.*, 2016, 4, 533-5.

[34] Kean, JM; Rao, S; Wang, M. Seroepidemiolgy of human polyomavirus. *PLoS Pathog*, 2009, 5, 1000363.

[35] Knowles, WA; Pipkin, P; Andrews, N. Population-based stufy of antibody to the human polyomaviruses BKV and JCV and the simian polyomavirus SV40. *J Med Virol*, 2003, 71, 115-23.

[36] Kappos, L; Wiend, H; Selmaj, K. Daclizumab HYP versus interferon beta 1-a in relapse remitting multiple sclerosis. *N Eng J Med.*, 2015, 373, 1418-28.

[37] Gorman, MP; Tillema, JM; Ciliax, AM; Guttmann, CR; Chitnis, T. Daclizumab use in patients with pediatric multiple sclerosis. *Arch Neurol*, 2012, 69, 78-81.

[38] Hauser, SL; Waubant, E; Arnold, DL. B-cell depletion with rituximab in relapsing-remitting multiple sclerosis. *N Engl J Med*, 2008, 358, 676, 676-88.

[39] Hauser, Sl; Bar-OR, A; Comi, G. OPERA 1 and OPERA 2 clinical investegation. Ocrelizumab verses interferon beta-1a in relapse remitting multiple sclerosis. *N Engl J Med*, 2017, 376, 221-34.

[40] Dale, RC; Brilot, F; Duffy, LV. Utility and safety of rituximab in pediatric autoimmune inflammatory CNS disease. *Neurology*, 2014, 2, 142-50.

[41] Tzaribachev, N; Koetter, I; Kuemmerle-Deschner, JB; Schedel, J. Rituximab for the treatment of refractory pediatric autoimmne disease: a case series. *Cases J*, 2009, 2, 66209.

[42] Chitnis, T; Waubant, E. B-cell depletion in children with neuormmunological conditions: a learning curve. *Neurology*, 2014, 2, 111-2.

[43] Carson, KR; Focosi, D; Major, EO. Monoclonal antibody associated progressive multifocal leucoencephalopathy in patients treated with rituximab, natalizumab, and efalizumab: a Review from the Research on Adverse Drug Events and Rports (RADAR) Project. *Lancet Oncol*, 2009, 10, 816-824.

[44] Chalkley, JJ; Berger, JR. Progressive multifocal leukoencephlopathy in multiple sclerosis. *Curr Neurol Neurosci*., 2013, 12, 408.

[45] Hauser, SL; Dawson, DM; Lehrich, JR; Beal, MF; Kevy, SV; Propper, RD; Mills, JA; Weiner, HL. Intesnive immunosuppression in progressive multiple scleroiss. A randomized, three-arm stufy of high-dose intravenous cyclophasphamide, plasma exchange, and ACTH. *N Engl J Med*., 1983, 4, 173-80.

[46] Weiner, HL; MAckin, GA; Orav, EJ. Intermittent cyclophospamide pulse therapy in progressive multple sclerois: final report of the Northeast Cooperative Multiple Sclerosis Treatment Group. *Neurology*, 1993 May, 43(5)910-8.

[47] Makhani, N; Gorman, MP; Branson, HM; Stazzone, L; Banwell, BL; Chitnis, T. Cyclophosphamide therapy in pediatric multiple sclerosis. *Neurology*, 2009, 2009, 72, 2076-82.

[48] Fragoso, YD; Alves-Leon, SV; Barreira, AA. Fingolimod prescribed for the treamnt of multiple sclerosis in patients younger than age 18. *Pediatr Neurol*, 2015, 263, 166-8.

[49] Chitnis, T; Ghezzi, A; Bajer-Kornek, B; Boyko, A; Giovannoni, G; Pohl, D. Pediatric multiple sclerosis escalation and emerging treatments. *Neurology*, 2016, 87, 103-9.

[50] Bomprezzi, R. Dimethyl Fumarate in the treatment of relapse-remitting multiple sclerosis: an overview. *Ther Adv Neurol Disord.*, 2015, 1, 20-30.

[51] Makhani, N; Schreiner, T. Oral dimethyl fumarate in chilren with multple sclerosis: A dual center study. *Pediatr Neurol.*, 2016, 57, 101-4.

[52] Jiwon, O; O'Conner, P. Teriflunomide in the treatment of multiple sclerosis: current evidence and future prospects. *Ther Adv Neurol Disord.*, 2014, 5, 239-52.

[53] Sorensen, P; Blinkenberg, M. The potential role of ocrelizumab in the treatment of multiple sclerosis: current evidence and future prospects. *Ther Adv Neurol Disord.*, 2016, 9, 44-52.

[54] Coles, A. Alemtuzumab therapy for multiple sclerosis. *J Neurotherapeutics.*, 2013, 1, 29-33.

[55] Etamadifar, M; Afzali, P; Abtahi, SH; Ramagopalan, SV; Nourian, SM; Murray, RT; Rereidan-Esfahani, M. Safety and efficacy of mitoxantrone in pediatric patients with aggressive multiple sclerosis. *Eur J paediatr Neurol.*, 2014, 2, 119-25.

[56] Chitnis, T; Tardieu, M; Amato, MP. International Pediatric MS sStudy Group Clincal Trials Summit: meeting report. *Neurology*, 2013, 80, 1161-8.

In: Multiple Sclerosis in Children … ISBN: 978-1-53612-979-3
Editors: H. Omar and J. Chalkley

Chapter 5

DISABILITY IN PATIENTS WITH PEDIATRIC-ONSET MULTIPLE SCLEROSIS

Ana C. Albuja*[*], *MD
Department of Neurology, Division of Child Neurology,
University of Kentucky, Lexington, KY, US

ABSTRACT

Pediatric onset multiple sclerosis (POMS) causes impairment in multiple domains, including physical, cognitive, and social. Physical disability is initially subtle and develops later in the course of the disease. Cognitive impairment is frequent and should be monitored closely. Fatigue and mood disorders occur as frequently in children as in adults with multiple sclerosis. All of these can have long-term effects on a child's quality of life, academic, and social functioning. When comparing patients with POMS to those with adult-onset disease of the same chronological age, those with POMS have poorer outcomes.

---

[*] Correspondence: Ana C. Albuja, MD. Chief Resident, Department of Neurology, Division of Child Neurology. 740 S. Limestone Room J422, Lexington, KY 40536-0234. E-mail: ana.albuja@uky.edu.

Keywords: pediatric onset multiple sclerosis, physical disability, cognitive disability, visual disability, quality of life

PHYSICAL DISABILITY

Currently, physical disability in patients with pediatric and adult-onset MS (AOMS) is most commonly evaluated using the Expanded Disability Status Scale (EDSS) [1]. This scale has limitations in the pediatric population. First, it is not very sensitive to evaluate disease severity because, as demonstrated in the studies described below, significant physical disability occurs decades after disease onset. Also, EDSS is a nonlinear, ordinal scale that has significant focus on disability secondary to problems with gait [1].

Given that the impairments in pediatric MS are usually subtle, hypothetically the use of dynamic measures as evaluated using the Multiple Sclerosis Functional Composite may be more sensitive. The goal of this scale is to quantify clinical information from areas usually affected in MS such as arm and leg function, and cognition. This is achieved by using 9-hole peg test, the 25-foot walk, and paced auditory serial addition task (PASAT). The problem with this test is that there is no normative data for the 25-foot walk in the pediatric population. It is also possible that this short distance is not sensitive to differentiate patients with POMS from healthy controls. The other challenge of following patients longitudinally with this dynamic measure is that there may be a change in the score for this scale as the child gets older and the ability to perform a task increases [1].

As of writing this chapter, the European Database for Multiple Sclerosis (EDMUS) has the largest database focused on outcome in patients with POMS. It includes 394 patients who were diagnosed with MS before 16 years of age, 30 of which were younger than 10 years at the time of onset. In addition, there were 1775 patients whose onset of MS symptoms occurred after 16 years of age. Almost 60% of these patients had received one or more disease modifying therapies (DMTs) including interferon beta, azathioprine, mitoxantrone, cyclophosphamide, and methotrexate. In most cases, patients with POMS reached an EDSS of 4 (limited walking ability but able to walk more than 500 meters without assistance or resting) nearly 20 years after their first attack. On the other hand, patients with AOMS reached this outcome approximately 8 years after their first attack. Interestingly, once patients reached an EDSS of 4, the time to reach and EDSS of 7 (ability to walk no more than 10 meters without resting using a wall or furniture for support) was on average 12.2 years for both groups [2].

Similar rates of disease progression were found in a population-based study in the United Kingdom. In this study, 111 patients who were younger than 18 years at the time of their first MS attack were compared to patients with AOMS. In this cohort, patients who did not experience a complete recovery after the first MS attack had a more rapid disease progression, as supported by a shorter median time to achieve an EDDSS of 4 (13.5 years in the group with incomplete recovery vs. 25.4 years in patients with complete recovery from their first attack) [3]. Similar findings were reported in the EDMUS [2].

In the EDMUS, pediatric patients advanced into secondary progressive MS (defined as progressive neurologic impairment, with or without discrete relapses) 10 years later than patients with AOMS (28.1 years after the first attack in POMS compared to 18.8 years in AOMS). However, patients with POMS were, on average, 10 years younger than those with AOMS by the time they developed secondary progressive MS (41 vs. 52 years) [2]. Other studies corroborate that, in POMS, longer disease duration is required before reaching irreversible disability or a secondary-progressive disease course as compared to AOMS. These studies also showed that, if comparing patients of the same chronological age, those whose disease onset occurred during childhood have poorer outcomes [4-6].

Visual Disability

When evaluating the anterior visual pathway, low-contrast letter acuity is used to assess function and optical coherence tomography (OCT) provides structural imaging. Studies have shown decreased low-contrast letter acuity scores as well as retinal nerve fiber layer (RNFL) thinning in patients with POMS and history of optic neuritis [7]. However, there is inconsistent data regarding the relationship between low-contrast letter acuity and retinal disease in patients with POMS without history of optic neuritis [8, 9].

Visual evoked potentials (VEP), somatosensory evoked potentials (SSEP) and brainstem auditory evoked potentials (BAEP) have been used primarily to identify asymptomatic areas of demyelination. A retrospective study of 85 pediatric patients with MS who underwent VEP, SSEP, and BAEP before their second clinical attack showed abnormal evoked potentials in 95% of the patients with visual symptoms, 57% of patients with sensory symptoms, and 46% of patients with brainstem symptoms [10].

These findings were corroborated on a prospective study with a smaller sample size [11].

While clinical recovery is usually complete, the data presented raise suspicion that anatomical abnormalities persist and that disease can still be quantified [2].

Cognitive Disability

Although multiple different definitions and diagnostic batteries for cognitive impairment are used in MS patients, cognitive difficulties are consistently reported in approximately one third of patients with POMS. A multicenter study performed in the US that included 187 patients with POMS defined cognitive impairment as test scores greater than 1 standard deviation below the published normative data for age, with deficiencies noted in at least one third of the total test domains. Cognitive impairment was found in 35% of patients with relapsing remitting MS and 18% of patients with clinically isolated syndrome. The most frequent deficits were in the areas of motor coordination (54%), visuomotor integration (51%), and speeded information processing (35%). Predictors of cognitive impairment included the diagnosis of MS (compared to patients with clinically isolated syndrome) and degree of disability in the EDSS [12].

An Italian multicenter study compared 63 patients with POMS with 57 matched healthy controls. Cognitive impairment was defined as scores falling below the 5th percentile (1.67 standard deviations –SD-) of healthy control performance in at least 3 tests. The population with MS had lower verbal and performance intelligence quotient (IQ) scores than healthy controls. Nineteen patients with MS met criteria for cognitive impairment. The areas that were more commonly affected were verbal ability (39-53%), visuospatial memory (18-56%), complex attention (28-50%), and executive function (41%). IQ was a predictor of cognitive impairment on logistic regression analysis. If IQ was labeled as a dependent variable, the only predictor of impaired cognition was younger age at the time of MS onset [13].

Till et al. studied 35 patients with POMS and 33 healthy controls. They found that patients with POMS had decreased functioning particularly in the areas of attention and processing speed (38%), visuomotor integration (23.5%), and expressive vocabulary (9.7%). The full and verbal IQ was significantly lower in the MS group compared to the control group. Among POMS patients, 14.3% had an IQ below 85 [14].

A study performed in the US in 37 patients with POMS found that 35.1% had cognitive impairment. This was defined as obtaining scores at least 1.5 SD below normative data in 2 or more cognitive tasks. Impairment was most frequently seen in complex attention (29.7%), object naming (18.9%), receptive language (13.5%), immediate recall of visual information (8.1%), and delayed recall of visual (11%) and verbal (18.9%) information. The greatest predictor of cognitive impairment was an elevated EDSS. The number of relapses was another prognostic factor.

Thirty-five percent of patients needed some type of accommodation in school [15].

There is limited information regarding the long-term cognitive outcome of patients with POMS [16]. Most longitudinal studies report gradual cognitive worsening, but its magnitude varies greatly between studies [17-22].

The Italian cohort evaluated patients at the time of enrollment, at 2, and 5 years. When comparing initial evaluation to 5 years, it was found that 56% of patients had declined, 19.8% of had stabilized, and 25% had improved their cognitive impairment index. The areas most likely to show decline were visual spatial learning and memory, verbal fluency, and expressive language [17, 18].

Till et al. studied changes in test scores over a period of 1 year in 28 patients with POMS and 26 controls using the Reliable Change Index. They categorized participants as demonstrating cognitive decline or improvement if there was a change in scores that exceeded the Reliable Change index in 3 or more tests. Seven (25%) of the patients with POMS had decline compared to 1 (4.6%) of the controls ($p < 0.05$) [21].

A cohort of 35 patients with POMS used growth curve modeling to evaluate changes in cognitive maturation. The authors showed that a younger age at the time of disease onset was associated with increased risk for cognitive decline in working memory and processing speed [19].

A multicenter study performed in the US with a sample of 62 pediatric patients with a formal diagnosis of MS and 5 patients with clinically isolated syndrome demonstrated that most patients remained stable when cognitive testing was repeated 1.6 years from the initial evaluation. Only 13% of the patients showed decline and 20% showed improvement in 2 or more tasks. It is possible that patient characteristics and assessment tools varied between this study and other studies described above, contributing to explain discrepancies in results [22].

In summary, cognitive impairment is frequent in pediatric patients with MS. Therefore, it is important to periodically evaluate cognitive maturation and to screen for the development of cognitive symptoms. With this said, a significant number of patients may show stable or improved cognitive function over the course of the disease [22].

DISABILITY DUE TO FATIGUE AND MOOD DISORDERS

Fatigue is a frequent complaint in pediatric and adult patients with MS. A study of 51 patients with POMS used the Pediatric QOL Inventory (PedsQL) Multidimensional Fatigue Scale to evaluate general, cognitive-, and sleep-related fatigue. It showed that 24% of patients had mild fatigue (1-2 SD below age-matched normative data) and 32% of the patients had severe fatigue (2 SD below age-matched normative data). Fifty-two percent of patients had cognitive fatigue, and 26% of patients had sleep-related fatigue.

Parents rated their children's fatigue as more severe than the child's self-report. They reported that their children had more cognitive fatigue (76%) than general and sleep-related fatigue (63% for each) [23]. Similar findings were reported in another study where 9 to 14% of POMS patients self-reported fatigue, compared to 23 to 39% of parents reporting fatigue in their children. In this particular study, there was a statistically significant relationship between fatigue and self-reported depressive symptoms. On the other hand, cognitive fatigue was associated with poor performance on cognitive tasks evaluating executive function, attention, memory, and processing speed [24]. In the Italian cohort, 20% of the 48 patients followed during a 5-year period met criteria for severe fatigue using the Fatigue Severity Scale [18]. These studies highlight the importance of screening for fatigue in neurologic follow-up visits because it is a disabling symptom that can affect school performance and can be treated in most cases.

In general, parents report higher prevalence of mood and behavioral disturbances in their children, as compared to self-reported rates by the child or adolescent [25]. In the Italian cohort, parents endorsed behavioral problems in 39% of POMS patients followed for a mean of 5 years. Psychiatric interviews revealed affective disturbances in 30% of children

[18]. In a study that used the Behavior Assessment System for Children, 2nd edition, 29% of parents rated their children with MS as positive for depression. In contrast, none of the parents of the healthy controls reported depression in their children [21]. Patients with cognitive dysfunction have increased risk for mood disorders [26]. There is also an association between behavioral issues and fatigue and lower full-scale IQ [27].

Quality of Life (QOL)

Two studies done in POMS patients used the PedsQL and showed lower health-related QOL in the first 2 years of disease [23, 28]. The school domain showed the greatest decrease in QOL, but physical and psychosocial well-being were also reduced when compared to controls. The total score in the PedsQL was 16 points lower in a cohort of 37 patients with POMS and 13 patients with clinically isolated syndrome as compared to their 12 siblings [used as controls) ($p = 0.004$). Likewise, when using the PedsQL parent proxy questionnaire, caregivers reported significantly reduced health-related QOL in their children with MS or clinically isolated syndrome compared to their healthy children (22-point difference, adjusted for age and sex, $p = 0.001$). There was a significant correlation between the patients' EDSS and PedsQL scores. A 1-point increase in the EDSS was correlated with a 4.5-point decrease in the total PedsQL score ($p = 0.014$) [28]. A study on self-reported fatigue, depression, and QOL in patients with POMS and AOMS showed comparable measurements in both groups [29].

Frequency of Relapses and Disability After Relapses

Patients with POMS usually have more frequent relapses in the first few years after disease onset as compared to their counterparts with

AOMS. For instance, a prospective study of 21 POMS and 110 AOMS patients showed that the annualized relapse rate (ARR) after 3 years was 1.1 in POMS compared to 0.4 in AOMS ($p = 0.001$) [30].

In addition to a greater relapse frequency, children and adolescents with MS often suffer more severe relapses compared to adults. However, they usually recover fully from them [30]. A retrospective cohort single-center study used a scoring system to classify patient's attacks as mild, moderate, or severe. The first group had functional system scores (FSS) of 0 to 1 in 3 or fewer domains, visual acuity better than 20/40, or EDSS between 0–1.5. The group with moderate disability had a FSS of 2 in 2 or fewer domains or an FSS of 1 in more than 3 domains, visual acuity between 20/40 and 20/190, or EDSS between 2 and 2.5. To classify as severe disability, a patient exceeded the parameters listed for moderate disability. Among 105 POMS patients, the initial attack was classified as mild in 16%, moderate in 32%, and severe in 53% [31]. In contrast, a study done previously in the same center showed that only 17% of initial attacks were classified as severe in AOMS patients. Interestingly, two-thirds of POMS patients, and only 46% of AOMS patients, reached complete recovery as defined by a FSS and an EDSS of 0 [32].

A study of pediatric and adult patients who presented with optic neuritis as a symptom of their first MS attack did not detect any difference in the severity of optic neuritis between adult and pediatric patients. Visual recovery at 1 year was also better in patients with POMS compared to AOMS [33].

In a Canadian study where patients with acquired demyelinating syndrome were followed prospectively, all children who were eventually diagnosed with MS recovered completely after their first attack ($n = 59$). Eighty-nine percent of these patients continued to have a normal neurological exam 4 or more years after the onset of symptoms [34]. There have been other studies performed in the UK and Iraq reporting that the majority of pediatric patients experience complete recovery after their first MS attack [3, 35, 36].

Effect of Disability on Academic and Social Functioning

Disability related to POMS can have a significant impact in the child's and adolescent's academic and social performance. In the Italian cohort, parents of one-third of children reported that cognitive problems negatively affected their children's school, daily, and social activities. Of 30 patients, 3 had a support teacher and 7 had to repeat a year in school. Forty-one percent of patients reported a negative effect of the disease on hobbies and sports. After 5 years of follow-up, cognitive decline was found to be associated with adverse outcomes on school achievements and social life [18].

A French study evaluated school performance in patients with POMS and other demyelinating diseases. They used grade retention as a validated measure of school performance. Grade retention happened in 151 (43.9%) of 344 patients during follow up (minimum 2 years). The risk for grade retention was higher in males, in children of families with a low socioeconomic status, in children who were older than 11 years at the time of onset, in children who had brainstem involvement or optic neuritis in the first attack, and in those who had irreversible disability after the first attack [37].

Conclusion

- Regarding physical disability, patients with POMS require longer disease duration before reaching irreversible disability or a secondary-progressive disease course as compared to AOMS. However, they are around 10 years younger by the time when they suffer irreversible disability.
- Cognitive impairment is frequent in POMS. For this reason, it is important to evaluate cognitive development and to screen for cognitive symptoms periodically. Nevertheless, a significant

number of patients may show stable or improved cognitive function over the course of the disease.

- Fatigue is as frequent in patients with POMS as in those with AOMS. It is important to screen for fatigue in neurological follow-up visits because it is a disabling symptom that can affect school performance and that can be treated in most cases.
- Approximately one third of the patients with POMS have mood disorders. Parents report higher prevalence of mood and behavioral disturbances in their children with POMS, as compared to self-reported rates by the child or adolescent. Cognitive dysfunction is associated with increased risk for mood disorders.
- Children and adolescents with MS often suffer more frequent and more severe relapses compared to adults. However, they usually recover fully from them.
- Disability related to POMS can have a significant impact in the child's and adolescent's academic performance. Cognitive problems can negatively affect activities of daily living, school performance, and social interactions.

REFERENCES

[1] Waldman A, Ness J, Pohl D, Simone IL, Anlar B, Amato MP, et al. Pediatric multiple sclerosis: Clinical features and outcome. *Neurology*. 2016;87(9 Suppl 2):S74-81.

[2] Renoux C, Vukusic S, Mikaeloff Y, Edan G, Clanet M, Dubois B, et al. Natural history of multiple sclerosis with childhood onset. *N Engl J Med*. 2007;356(25):2603-13.

[3] Harding KE, Liang K, Cossburn MD, Ingram G, Hirst CL, Pickersgill TP, et al. Long-term outcome of paediatric-onset multiple sclerosis: a population-based study. *J Neurol Neurosurg Psychiatry*. 2013;84(2):141-7.

[4] Boiko A, Vorobeychik G, Paty D, Devonshire V, Sadovnick D. Early onset multiple sclerosis: a longitudinal study. *Neurology*. 2002;59(7):1006-10.

[5] Simone IL, Carrara D, Tortorella C, Liguori M, Lepore V, Pellegrini F, et al. Course and prognosis in early-onset MS: comparison with adult-onset forms. *Neurology*. 2002;59(12):1922-8.

[6] Ghezzi A, Pozzilli C, Liguori M, Marrosu MG, Milani N, Milanese C, et al. Prospective study of multiple sclerosis with early onset. *Mult Scler*. 2002;8(2):115-8.

[7] Waldman AT, Hiremath G, Avery RA, Conger A, Pineles SL, Loguidice MJ, et al. Monocular and binocular low-contrast visual acuity and optical coherence tomography in pediatric multiple sclerosis. *Mult Scler Relat Disord*. 2013;3(3):326-34.

[8] Yeh EA, Weinstock-Guttman B, Lincoff N, Reynolds J, Weinstock A, Madurai N, et al. Retinal nerve fiber thickness in inflammatory demyelinating diseases of childhood onset. *Mult Scler*. 2009;15(7): 802-10.

[9] Yilmaz U, Gucuyener K, Erin DM, Yazar Z, Gurkas E, Serdaroglu A, et al. Reduced retinal nerve fiber layer thickness and macular volume in pediatric multiple sclerosis. *J Child Neurol*. 2012;27(12):1517-23.

[10] Pohl D, Rostasy K, Treiber-Held S, Brockmann K, Gartner J, Hanefeld F. Pediatric multiple sclerosis: detection of clinically silent lesions by multimodal evoked potentials. *J Pediatr*. 2006;149(1):125-7.

[11] Voitenkov V, Skripchenko N, Klimkin A. Visual pathways involvement in clinically isolated syndrome in children. *Int J Ophthalmol*. 2015;8(2):382-4.

[12] Julian L, Serafin D, Charvet L, Ackerson J, Benedict R, Braaten E, et al. Cognitive impairment occurs in children and adolescents with multiple sclerosis: results from a United States network. *J Child Neurol*. 2013;28(1):102-7.

[13] Amato MP, Goretti B, Ghezzi A, Lori S, Zipoli V, Portaccio E, et al. Cognitive and psychosocial features of childhood and juvenile MS. *Neurology*. 2008;70(20):1891-7.

[14] Till C, Ghassemi R, Aubert-Broche B, Kerbrat A, Collins DL, Narayanan S, et al. MRI correlates of cognitive impairment in childhood-onset multiple sclerosis. *Neuropsychology*. 2011;25(3): 319-32.

[15] MacAllister WS, Belman AL, Milazzo M, Weisbrot DM, Christodoulou C, Scherl WF, et al. Cognitive functioning in children and adolescents with multiple sclerosis. *Neurology*. 2005;64(8):1422-5.

[16] Marin SE, Banwell BB, Till C. Cognitive trajectories in 4 patients with pediatric-onset multiple sclerosis: serial evaluation over a decade. *J Child Neurol*. 2013;28(12):1577-86.

[17] Amato MP, Goretti B, Ghezzi A, Lori S, Zipoli V, Moiola L, et al. Cognitive and psychosocial features in childhood and juvenile MS: two-year follow-up. *Neurology*. 2010;75(13):1134-40.

[18] Amato MP, Goretti B, Ghezzi A, Hakiki B, Niccolai C, Lori S, et al. Neuropsychological features in childhood and juvenile multiple sclerosis: five-year follow-up. *Neurology*. 2014;83(16):1432-8.

[19] Hosseini B, Flora DB, Banwell BL, Till C. Age of onset as a moderator of cognitive decline in pediatric-onset multiple sclerosis. *J Int Neuropsychol Soc*. 2014;20(8):796-804.

[20] MacAllister WS, Christodoulou C, Milazzo M, Krupp LB. Longitudinal neuropsychological assessment in pediatric multiple sclerosis. *Dev Neuropsychol*. 2007;32(2):625-44.

[21] Till C, Racine N, Araujo D, Narayanan S, Collins DL, Aubert-Broche B, et al. Changes in cognitive performance over a 1-year period in children and adolescents with multiple sclerosis. *Neuropsychology*. 2013;27(2):210-9.

[22] Charvet LE, O'Donnell EH, Belman AL, Chitnis T, Ness JM, Parrish J, et al. Longitudinal evaluation of cognitive functioning in pediatric multiple sclerosis: report from the US Pediatric Multiple Sclerosis Network. *Mult Scler*. 2014;20(11):1502-10.

In: Multiple Sclerosis in Children … ISBN: 978-1-53612-979-3
Editors: H. Omar and J. Chalkley

Chapter 6

ALTERNATIVE TREATMENTS IN PEDIATRIC MULTIPLE SCLEROSIS

Roman M. Kassa*, MD, PhD
Department of Neurology, University of Kentucky,
Lexington, KY, US

ABSTRACT

Symptom management is an integral part of the care of patients with multiple sclerosis. Complementary and alternative treatments have been mostly used for the management of symptoms in this patient population. The purpose of this paper is to review the literature on the various treatment modalities and available data supporting their use.

Keywords: complementary medicine, alternative medicine, pediatric multiple sclerosis

---

* Corresponding Author E-mail: roman.kassa@uky.edu.

INTRODUCTION

Long term treatment of multiple sclerosis has been largely divided into two arms, which go hand in hand: disease-modifying therapies and symptom management. Therapies which are not mainstream and are used in lieu of conventional treatments are referred to as alternative interventions, and when used in conjunction with prevailing treatment modalities are called complementary medical therapies. Complementary and alternative medicine (CAM) is, by definition, not part of conventional medicine due to insufficient evidence regarding safety and efficacy. CAM is mostly used to treat common multiple sclerosis-associated symptoms such as fatigue, spasticity, stiffness, pain, tremor, imbalance, depression, cognitive impairment, insomnia, and bladder and bowel dysfunction. There is heterogeneity of data and paucity of solid scientific evidence available on the efficacy and safety of treatments available for these symptoms in patients with multiple sclerosis in general and the pediatric population, in particular.

As in the adult population, fatigue is a predominant symptom in pediatric multiple sclerosis patients. A study examining the overall quality of life of patients with multiple sclerosis with age range of 9 to 17 years of age showed that 56% of patients self-reported fatigue, 52% cognitive difficulties, 28% emotional problems and 26% sleep problems [1]. Both self-reported and parent proxy-reported scores reflecting health-related quality of life were found to be substantially reduced among children with multiple sclerosis and clinically isolated syndrome compared to subjects with no neurological problems [2]. Moreover, children with multiple sclerosis also had worse self-reported emotional and school functioning compared to patients with neuromuscular disorders [2].

Based on the classification system recognized by the National Center for Complementary and Alternative Medicine, there are at least five broad categories of CAM commonly used by patients with multiple sclerosis. These include manipulative and body-based therapies (Chinese acupuncture, electroacupuncture, hippotherapy, massage therapy, movement therapies, reflexology, yoga), mind-body therapies (biofeedback, relaxation, hypnosis, meditation, mindfulness-based training, music therapy), energy healing therapies (magnetic therapy, neural therapy), biologically-based therapies (herbs such as cannabis and *Ginkgo biloba*, bee venom, chelation therapy, hyperbaric oxygen, minerals, Padma 28, special diets, nonvitamin nonmineral natural products such as fish oil, alpha lipoic acid, primrose oil, flaxseed oil) and alternative medical systems (homeopathic treatment, naturopathy, traditional healers) [3]. An overall prevalence of CAM use ranging from 33% to 80% is reported in adult multiple sclerosis patients [4, 5]. A small study consisting of thirty-five adult patients with diagnosis of multiple sclerosis at least one year prior to enrollment found that 77.1% of patients used CAM in the previous year [3], a prevalence that is almost twice as much as that reported in the general US population [6]. Interestingly, this study also showed that about 11.8% of children in the general population had used some type of CAM in the prior 12 months based on parent proxy reports.

Among children with neurologic disorders, a cross-sectional study of a population of patients with the age of 2-18 years in an outpatient neurology clinic with brain injury, epilepsy, headache and neuromuscular diseases revealed that 44% used at least one type of CAM [7]. Another study reported that significantly more children aged 3-17 years of age with common neurological conditions comprising migraine headache, non-migrainous headache and seizure used CAM compared to children without these conditions, i.e., 24% vs 12.6%, respectively [8]. However, scientific studies on the prevalence of CAM use in the pediatric population with multiple sclerosis are lacking.

The American Academy of Neurology (AAN) released the most comprehensive literature review from 1970 to September 2013 and evidence-based practice guidelines regarding the use of CAM in multiple sclerosis were published in March 2014. Main questions addressed included whether CAM use interferes with disease-modifying therapies, possible serious side effects or worsening of multiple sclerosis with their use, and efficacy in reducing multiple-sclerosis-associated symptoms as well as preventing relapses and disability.

Level A recommendations were found for effectiveness of short term oral cannabis extract use for subjective spasticity symptoms and pain which is not of central neuropathic origin. Level B recommendations were made regarding use of oromucosal cannabinoid spray for spasticity, pain, and urinary frequency as well as magnetic therapy for fatigue reduction. This also included the use of tetrahydrocannabinol (THC) for subjective spasticity symptoms and pain. Level C recommendations included use of *Gingko biloba* for fatigue, and reflexology for multiple-sclerosis related paresthesia. Analysis of the data was insufficient to determine whether CAM use is associated with worsening of multiple sclerosis or if they interfere with disease-modifying therapies [9]. Of note, these recommendations are based on studies in the adult population with multiple sclerosis. Thus, careful consideration and caution should be exercised when trying to extrapolate these recommendations to the pediatric population. Below are brief discussions regarding selected CAM therapies including their proposed mechanism of action and data regarding therapeutic effect or lack thereof in the management of largely multiple sclerosis-associated symptoms.

CANNABIS

The major cannabinoids of the cannabis plant are delta-9-THC and cannabidiol (CBD). Different forms of cannabis have been utilized in patients with multiple sclerosis for symptom management and include standardized oral cannabis extract containing THC and CBD, synthetic THC, oromucosal cannabinoid spray, and smoked cannabis.

It has been proposed that the endogenous cannabinoid system may modulate tremor and spasticity, and that agonists of the receptor CB1, may have therapeutic effects in the suppression of spasticity and tremor [10]. Data regarding the pharmacologic characteristics of cannabinoids suggest that THC directly modulates the activity of cannabinoid receptors- CB1, CB2 and putative CB2-like receptors. Furthermore, studies in mice with chronic relapsing experimental allergic encephalomyelitis, which is an autoimmune model of multiple sclerosis, have shown that cannabinoid receptor agonists such as THC quantitatively improved tremor and spasticity [11].

Oral Cannabis Extract and Synthetic THC

Based on class I studies, oral cannabis extract was found to be effective in reducing patient-reported symptoms of spasticity and pain in primary progressive, relapsing remitting and secondary progressive multiple sclerosis patients [12, 13] (Level A). Subjective benefit from this therapy is possibly maintained over a 12-month period (Level C). The AAN guideline of 2014 regarding CAM use in multiple sclerosis patients also indicates that physicians might also offer THC for patient-reported spasticity symptoms and pain which is not central neuropathic pain [12] (Level B). It can be offered to patients with all types of multiple sclerosis. In parallel to oral cannabis extract, benefit from synthetic THC use in terms of self-reported spasticity and pain is also possibly sustained for 1 year [14] (Level C). Both oral cannabis extracts and THC are probably ineffective for improving objective spasticity measures short term (i.e., 15 weeks) as well as controlling multiple sclerosis-related tremor and bladder symptoms [12] (Level B).

Oromucosal Cannabinoid Spray and Smoked Cannabis

The principal active components of oromucosal cannabinoid spray are THC and CBD, with each spray delivering about 1:1 ratio. It is not FDA approved, but has received regulatory approval in other countries including UK, Canada, Germany, Denmark, Sweden, Spain, Czech Republic, and support is critical for the individual with multiple sclerosis, their family and caretakers, and their friends.

Keywords: multiple sclerosis, pediatric, relationships, family, friends

Introduction

When children and adolescents are diagnosed with multiple sclerosis (MS), not only are they learning to live with a chronic disease but their family and friends are undergoing significant adjustments as well. MS is defined as a progressive disease that may or may not have relapses [1]. A relapse is unpredictable as to when it may occur and how it may manifest [1]. The unpredictability of the disease contributes the psychosocial stress that MS can cause. A relapse may involve symptoms such as a change in sensation, pain, cognition, balance, strength, coordination, vision, and bladder control [1]. Although MS does not occur as commonly in children and adolescents as it does in adults, there are still an estimated 8,000-10,000 children and adolescents under 18 years of age in the United States with a diagnosis of MS [2]. In addition, another 10,000-15,000 children and adolescents have experienced at least one symptom that is suggestive of MS [2].

The course of the disease in children and adolescents often differs from that in adults. Unfortunately, children tend to experience more frequent relapses than adults with early MS [2]. Also, increasing evidence suggests that while the disease course is often slower in children with MS, they may be more prone to significant disability that accumulates at an early age when compared with adult onset MS [2]. Depending on the severity of illness and the frequency of relapse, pediatric MS can affect all aspects of a child or adolescent's life. Affected areas include family relationships, relationships with peers, self-esteem, and academic performance [2]. Children and adolescents with severe disease may have decreased mobility and even become dependent on parents or other caregivers for activities of daily living. Each individual with MS is affected differently and the effects

Poland. Studies show that it has probable effectiveness for improving subjective spasticity symptoms over 6 weeks, central neuropathic pain over 5 weeks, and daily bladder frequency over 10 weeks [15-17] (Level B). In contrast, oromucosal cannabinoid spray is probably ineffective in the treatment of multiple sclerosis-related tremor over 15 weeks [18] (Level C).

Studies regarding the use of smoked cannabis for symptom management in multiple sclerosis were inconclusive [9]. It is noteworthy that standardized oral cannabis extracts which are not commercially available were used in the above clinical trials. Thus, careful deliberation regarding the safety and efficacy of the nonregulated forms of the different formulations is recommended by the AAN guideline authors. Another primary concern is central side effects with the use of cannabinoids such as dizziness, somnolence, poor concentration and memory problems [9].

LOW-FAT DIET WITH OMEGA-3 FATTY ACID SUPPLEMENTATION

Epidemiological studies from the 1950s suggested a strong association between low fish, high meat and high dairy products diet and increased incidence of multiple sclerosis [19]. It was postulated that frequency of multiple sclerosis was associated with calculated fat consumption of different populations. A large non-randomized, prospective study of adult multiple sclerosis patients spanning over 34 years was undertaken and reported a correlation with low saturated fat content and reduction in relapse, severity, disability, and mortality [20].

The authors of the AAN guideline reviewed the literature and recommend that clinicians may counsel patients that low fat diet with fish oil is probably ineffective for preventing relapses, fatigue, disability, radiological evidence of disease burden, or improving quality of life [21, 22] (Level B).

GINKGO BILOBA

At present, there are no effective therapies for the treatment of multiple sclerosis-associated cognitive impairment. *Ginkgo biloba* is an herb used in traditional medicine for millennia of years and is native to China. It is one of the most commonly used herbal medicines worldwide. The extract from this herb contains phytochemicals that target free-radical scavenging, have anti-inflammatory activity and improve blood flow, in addition to cholinesterase inhibition [23]. Studies suggest that *Ginkgo biloba* may improve memory and cognition in patients with Alzheimer's disease [24, 25], and thus the interest in exploring its effectiveness in the treatment of multiple-sclerosis associated dementia.

In two class I studies, no significant improvement in cognition with use of this herb was found in patients with multiple sclerosis [26, 27]. On the other hand, 240mg/day of *Gingko biloba* taken over 4 weeks is possibly effective in reducing fatigue in patients with multiple sclerosis compared to placebo [28]. The AAN guideline also indicates that interaction between *Gingko biloba* and other supplements is of clinical concern.

It has been hypothesized that one of the main effects of *Ginkgo biloba* is to increase blood flow and microcirculation through increased erythrocyte flexibility and reducing blood viscosity [29, 30]. Effect of this herb's extract on anticoagulation has been controversial, with multiple case reports of spontaneous bleeding after its use [31-33]. The data is heterogenous with concurrent use of anticoagulation or antiplatelet agents in several cases. A systematic review and meta-analysis of randomized controlled trials evaluating the impact the herb extract as single therapy versus placebo based on parameters of homeostasis did not reveal a higher risk of bleeding with the use of a standardized extract [34]. When discussing use of this herb by patients with multiple sclerosis, one also needs to consider possible interaction with antiplatelet or antithrombotic agent that they might be on.

REFLEXOLOGY

Reflexology is based on the belief that each body organ is represented in specific areas of the hands and feet, with massage of these sites leading to therapeutic benefit. It has been reported that reflexology led to significant improvement in pain in patients with cancer, headache and chronic pain associated with herniated disc [35, 36].

The AAN guideline indicates that reflexology is possibly effective for reducing multiple sclerosis-associated paresthesia over 11 weeks (Level C) and no significant safety concerns were found in the studies reviewed.

MINDFULNESS OF MOVEMENT AND TAI CHI

Mindfulness of Movement and Tai Chi

Some studies have shown that exercises that have a mindful and introspective aspect have significant impact on symptom improvement in patients with MS. The principle of mindfulness of movement in Tai Chi involves a steady awareness of whether breathing is deep or shallow, posture is aligned or not, sense of mind-body connection in terms of mental preparation of movement, and sense of whether there is muscular tension [37]. A pilot study examining the effect of mindfulness, with additional focus also on flow of movement and compassionate acceptance of one's own body, on symptom management in patients with multiple sclerosis showed a significant consistent pattern of improvement and less decline compared to the control group. Symptoms rated included walking distance, balance, bladder dysfunction, paresthesia, fatigue, and pain. This effect was also maintained at 3 month follow up [37]. Furthermore, improved walking speed over 25 feet by 21%, decreased spasticity with increase in hamstring flexibility by 28%, as well as amelioration in mental health and social functioning was found in Tai Chi-trained multiple sclerosis patients after an 8-week program [38].

Cooling Therapy

Fatigue is one of the most common symptoms experienced by patients with multiple sclerosis, considered by many to be the most debilitating, and is reported in at least 60-70% of individuals [39]. Central motor conduction block in response to temperature in partially demyelinated axons has been implicated as the mechanism for clinical worsening with elevated body temperature [40], and has been quantified by magnetic stimulation studies [41]. Cooling therapy utilizing a cooling vest resulting in lowering of body temperature by about 0.5-1°C showed significant improvement in the severity and impact of fatigue in the treated group [42]. Another small study with a cooling suit for the head and upper body which drops core body temperature by 0.1-1°C showed reduction in fatigue and improvement in the quality of life [43]. Moreover, a cooling device with thigh cuffs which decreases local skin temperature by 4-6°C over 1 hour showed significant improvement in muscle strength of the legs, 25-feet timed walking test, manual dexterity assessed via the 9-Hole Peg Test and cognition as evaluated by the Paced Auditory Serial Addition Test every 3 seconds [40].

Low Dose Naltrexone

Modulation of a biological pathway within the endogenous opioid system involving an opioid growth factor, methionine enkephalin, and its receptor via the administration of exogenous opioid antagonists has been shown to modulate replication of activated astrocytes and T lymphocytes [44,45]. Interestingly, administration of low dose naltrexone for a period of at least 10 months showed reduction of fatigue and improved quality of life in 60% and 75%, respectively, of patients with both relapsing remitting and secondary progressive multiple sclerosis and mean disease duration of 10 years [46]. Side effects such as nightmares and insomnia were reported in this study. Data so far also indicate that this treatment is nontoxic with no significant adverse effects [47].

References

[1] MacAlliter WS, Christodoulou C, Troxell R, Milazzo M, Block P, Preston TE, Bender HA, Belman A, Kurpp LB. Fatigue and quality of life in pediatric multiple sclerosis. *Mult Scler* 2009;15(12):502-8.

[2] Mowry EM, Julian LJ, Im-Wang S, Chabas D, Galvin AJ, Strober JB, Waubant E. Health-related quality of life is reduced in pediatric multiple sclerosis. *Pediatr Neurol* 2010;43(2):97-102.

[3] Masullo L, Papas MA, Cotugna N, Baker S, Mahoney L, Trabulsi J. Complementary and alternative medicine use and nutrient intake among individuals with multiple sclerosis in the United States. *J Community Health* 2015;40:153-60.

[4] Apel A, Greim B, König N, Zettl UK. Frequency of current utilization of complementary and alternative medicine by patients with multiple sclerosis. *J Neurol* 2006;253(10):13316.

[5] Schwartz S, Knorr C, Geiger H, Flachenecker P. Complementary and alternative medicine for multiple sclerosis. *Mult Scler* 2008;14(8):1113-9.

[6] Barnes PM, Bloom B, Nahin RL. Complementary and alternative medicine use among adults and children: United States, 2007. *Natl Health Stat Report* 2008;12:1-23.

[7] Soo I, Mah JK, Barlow K, Hamiwka L, Wirrell E. Use of complementary and alternative medical therapies in a pediatric neurology clinic. *Can J Neurol Sci* 2005;32:524-8.

[8] Treat L, Liesinger J, Ziegenfuss JY, Humeniuk K, Prasad K, Tilburt JC. Patterns of complementary and alternative medicine use in children with common neurological conditions. *Glob Adv Health Med* 2014;3(1):18-24.

[9] Yadav V, Bever C Jr, Bowen J, Bowling A, Weinstock-Guttman B, Cameron M, Bourdette D, Gronseth GS, Narayanaswami P.

Summary of evidence-based guideline: complementary and alternative medicine in multiple sclerosis: report of the guideline development subcommittee of the American Academy of Neurology. *Neurology* 2014;82(12):1083-92.

[10] Pertwee RG. Pharmacology of cannabinoid receptor ligands. *Curr Med Chem* 1999;6(8):635-64.

[11] Baker D, Pryce G, Croxford JL, Brown P, Pertwee RG, Huffman JW, Layward L. Cannabinoids control spasticity and tremor in a multiple sclerosis model. *Nature* 2000;40496773):84-7.

[12] Zajicek J, Fox P, Sanders H, Wright D, Vickery J, Nunn A, Thompson A, UK MS Research Group. Cannabinoids for treatment of spasticity and other symptoms related to multiple sclerosis (CAMS study): multicentre randomized placebo-controlled trial. *Lancet* 2003;362(9395):1517-26.

[13] Zajicek JP, Hobart JC, Slade A, Barnes D, Mattison PG, MUSEC Research Group. Multiple sclerosis and extract of cannabis: results of the MUSEC trial. *J Neurol Neurosurg Psychiatry* 2012;83(11): 1125-32.

[14] Zajicek JP, Sanders HP, Wright DE, Vickery PJ, Ingram WM, Reilly SM, Nunn AJ, Teare LJ, Fox PJ, Thompson AJ. Cannabinoids in multiple sclerosis (CAMS) study: safety and efficacy data for 12 months follow up. *J Neurol Neurosurg Psychiatry* 2005;76(12): 1664-9.

[15] Wade DT, Makela P, Robson P, House H, Bateman C. Do cannabis-based medicinal extracts have general or specific effects on symptoms in multiple sclerosis? A double-blind, randomized, placebo-controlled study on 160 patients. *Mult Scler* 2004;10(4):434-41.

[16] Rog DJ, Nurmikko TJ, Friede T, Young CA. Randomized, controlled trial of cannabis-based medicine in central pain in multiple sclerosis. *Neurology* 2005;65(6):812-9.

[17] Kavia RB, De Ridder D, Constantinescu CS, Stott CG, Fowler CJ. Randomized controlled trial of Sativex to treat detrusor overactivity in multiple sclerosis. *Mult Scler* 2010;16(11):1349-59.

[18] Collin C, Ehler E, Waberzinek G, Alsindi Z, Davies P, Powell K, Notcutt W, O'Leary C, Ratcliffe S, Nováková I, Zapletalova O, Piková J, Ambler Z. A double-blind, randomized, placebo-controlled, parallel-group study of Sativex, in subjects with symptoms of spasticity due to multiple sclerosis. *Neurol Res* 2010; 32(5):451-9.

[19] Swank RL, Lerstad O, Strøm A, Backer J. Multiple sclerosis in rural Norway- its geographic and occupational incidence in relation to nutrition. *N Engl J Med* 1952:246:721-8.

[20] Swank RL, Dugan BB. Effect of low saturated fat diet in early and late cases of multiple sclerosis. *Lancet* 1990;336:37-9.

[21] Bates D, Cartlidge NE, French JM, Jackson MJ, Nightingale S, Shaw DA, Smith S, Woo E, Hawkins SA, Millar JH. A double-blind controlled trial of long chain n-3 polyunsaturated fatty acids in the treatment of multiple sclerosis. *J Neurol Neruosurg Psychiatry* 1989;52(1):18-22.

[22] Weinstock-Guttman B, Baier M, Park Y, Feichter J, Lee-Kwen P, Gallagher E, Venkatraman J, Meksawan K, Deinehart S, Pendergast D, Awad AB, Ramanathan M, Munschauer F, Rudick R. Low fat dietary intervention with ω-3 fatty acid supplementation in multiple sclerosis patients. *Prostaglandins Leukot Essent Fatty Acids* 2005;73(5):397-404.

[23] Wightman EL. Potential benefits of phytochemicals against Alzheimer's disease. *Proc Nutr Soc* 2017;76(2):106-12.

[24] Oken BS, Storzbach DM, Kaye JA. The efficacy of Ginkgo biloba on cognitive function in Alzheimer disease. *Arch Neurol* 1998;55: 1409-15.

[25] Diamond BJ, Johnson SK, Torsney K, Morodan J, Prokop BJ, Davidek D, Kramer P. Complementary and alternative medicines in the treatment of dementia: An evidence-based review. *Drugs Aging* 2003;20(13):981-98.

[26] Lovera J, Bagert B, Smoot K, Morris CD, Frank R, Bogardus K, Wild K, Oken B, Whitham R, Bourdette D. Gingko biloba for the improvement of cognitive performance in multiple sclerosis: a randomized, placebo-controlled trial. *Mult Scler* 2007;13(3):376-85.

[27] Lovera JF, Kim E, Heriza E, Fitzpatrick M, Hunziker J, Turner AP, Adams J, Stover T, Sangeorzan A, Sloan M, Howieson D, Wild K, Haselkom J, Bourdette D. Gingko biloba does not improve cognitive function in MS: a randomized placebo-controlled trial. *Neurology* 2012;79(12):1278-84.

[28] Johnson SK, Diamond BJ, Rausch S, Kaufman M, Shiflett SC, Graves L. The effect of Gingko biloba on functional measures in multiple sclerosis: a pilot randomized controlled trial. *Explore* (NY) 2006;2(1):19-24.

[29] DeFeudis FV, Drieu K. Gingko biloba extract (EGb 761) and CNS functions: basic studies and clinical applications. *Curr Drug Targets* 2000;1(1):25-8.

[30] Diamond BJ, Shiflett SC, Feiwel N, Matheis RJ, Noskin O, Richards JA, Schoenberger NE. Gingko biloba extract: mechanisms and clinical indications. *Arch Phys Med Rehabil* 2000;81(5):668-78.

[31] MacVie OP, Harney BA. Vitreous haemorrhage associated with Gingko biloba use in a patient with age related macular disease. *Br J Ophthalmol* 2005;89(10):1378-9.

[32] Pedroso JL, Henriques Aquino CC, Escórcio Bezerra ML, Baiense RF, Suarez MM, Dutra LA, Braga-Neto P, Povoas Barsottini OG. Gingko biloba and cerebral bleeding: a case report and critical review. *Neurologist* 2011;17(2):89-90.

[33] Carlile PV. Unexplained alveolar hemorrhage associated with Gingko and ginseng use. *J Bronchology Interv Pulmonol* 2015;22(2):170-2.

[34] Kellermann AJ, Kloft C. Is there a risk of bleeding associated with standardized *Gingko biloba* extract therapy? A systematic review and meta-analysis. *Phramacotherapy* 2011;31(5);490-502.

[35] Launsø L, Brendstrup E, Arnberg S. An exploratory study of reflexological treatment for headache. *Altern Ther Health Med* 1999;5(3):57-65.

[36] Stephenson NL, Weinrich SP, Tavakoli AS. The effects of foot reflexology on anxiety and pain in patients with breast and lung cancer. *Oncol Nurs Forum* 2000;27(1):67-72.

[37] Mills N, Allen J. Mindfulness of movement as a coping strategy in multiple sclerosis. *Gen Hosp Psychiatry* 2000;22(6);425-31.

[38] Husted C, Pham L, Hekking A, Niederman R. Improving quality of life for people with chronic conditions: the example of t'ai chi and multiple sclerosis. *Altern Ther Health Med* 1999;5(5):70-4.

[39] Lerdal A, Cellus EG, Krupp L, Dahl AA. A prospective study of patterns of fatigue in multiple sclerosis. *Eur J Neurol* 2007;14(12):1338-43.

[40] Meyer-Heim A, Rothmaier M, Weder M, Kool J, Schenk P, Kesselring J. Advanced lightweight cooling-garment technology: functional improvements in thermosensitive patients with multiple sclerosis. *Mult Scler* 2007;13(2):232-7.

[41] Humm AM, Beer S, Kool J, Magistris MR, Kesselring J, Rosler KM. Quantification of Uhthoff's phenomenon in multiple sclerosis: a magnetic stimulation study. *Clin Neurophysiol* 2004;115(11):2493-2501.

[42] Ozkan Tuncay F, Mollaoglu M. Effect of the cooling suit method applied to individuals with multiple sclerosis on fatigue and activities of daily living. *J Clin Nurs* 2017; doi: 10.1111/jocn.13788.

[43] Flensner G, Lindencrona C. The cooling-suit: case studies of its influence on fatigue among eight individuals with multiple sclerosis. *J Adv Nurs* 2002;37(6):541-50.

[44] Zagon IS, McLaughlin PJ. Gene-peptide relationships in the developing rat brain: the response of preproenkephalin mRNA and [Met^5]-enkephalin to acute opioid antagonist (naltrexone) exposure. *Mol Brain Res* 1995;33:111-20.

[45] Rahn KA, McLaughlin PJ, Zagon IS. Prevention and diminished expression of experimental autoimmune encephalomyelitis by low dose naltrexone (LDN) or opioid growth factor (OGF) for an extended period: Therapeutic implications for multiple sclerosis. *Brain Res* 2011;1381:243-53.

[46] Turel AP, Oh KH, Zagon IS, McLaughlin PJ. Low dose naltrexone for treatment of multiple sclerosis: A retrospective chart review of safety and tolerability. *J Clin Psychopharmacol* 2015;35(5):609-11.

[47] Ludwig MD, Turel AP, Zagon IS, McLaughlin PJ. Long-term treatment with low dose naltrexone maintains stable health in patients with multiple sclerosis. *Mult Scler J Exp Transl Clin* 2016; 29(2):2055217316672242.

In: Multiple Sclerosis in Children … ISBN: 978-1-53612-979-3
Editors: H. Omar and J. Chalkley

Chapter 7

ADOLESCENTS AND MULTIPLE SCLEROSIS: THE PSYCHOLOGICAL EFFECTS OF DIAGNOSIS

Amy L. Burnett, MSN, APRN*
Division of Adolescent Medicine and Young Parent Programs, Kentucky Clinic, Department of Pediatrics, Kentucky Children's Hospital, University of Kentucky College of Medicine, Lexington, KY, US

ABSTRACT

Multiple sclerosis (MS) is not a common diagnosis found in the pediatric population. Only 5% of those diagnosed with MS are in the pediatric age category. Due to the stage of development and impaired coping skills, adolescents are at high risk of negative outcomes when given an MS diagnosis. It is imperative for these teens to have strong

---

* Corresponding Author Address: Amy Burnett, APRN. Department of Pediatrics, Division of Adolescent Medicine. 740 S. Limestone, Lexington, KY 40536. E-mail: amy.burnett1@uky.edu.

positive support from parents, peers, school officials, and medical providers to ensure a good outcome. This chapter explores potential negative psychosocial outcomes in adolescents with MS and the interventions shown to be effective in prevention.

Keywords: multiple sclerosis, adolescence, pediatric, psychological, mental health

Introduction

In what should be the most fun and care-free time in one's life, the diagnosis of a chronic disease in the adolescent years can be devastating, both physically and emotionally. This is a time of perceived invincibility, which makes a serious diagnosis, such a Multiple Sclerosis (MS), very difficult for a teenager to accept. Only 5% of all MS diagnoses occur in pediatric patients [1]. Due to the rarity of adolescent MS diagnoses, there has not been a great deal of research performed regarding the psychosocial effects that this diagnosis carries [1]. Even with a lack of research, it is assumed that such a significant diagnosis would profoundly affect a teenager emotionally and socially. This article aims to explore the psychosocial effects of MS on the adolescent population and what can be done to help teenagers cope with these issues in a healthy way.

Multiple Sclerosis and the Adolescent

According to Eric Erikson, the adolescent years are a time of identity development [2]. During this bridge from childhood to adulthood, adolescents are trying to determine who they are and who they want to become [2]. The teenage years are also a time of rapid brain development and growth [3]. The myelination in the developing central nervous system (CNS) occurs during this time, which is thought to play a large role in the physical and cognitive difficulties faced with adolescent onset MS [4]. A diagnosis such as MS does not have to lead to dysfunction in this age group [4]. It takes a team approach, involving the patient, family, friends, and healthcare providers, to ensure the best outcomes for adolescents with an MS diagnosis.

It is estimated that around 50% of adolescents diagnosed with MS will have some level of cognitive decline [5]. Due to MS being a demyelinating CNS process, it can have significant impacts on the individual when it develops during the time of rapid brain myelination [4]. With a decrease in cognitive functioning, there can be an associated decrease in the ability to process information and employ adaptive skills vital for healthy coping [5]. It has been noted that higher IQ's are a protective factor for mental health during childhood [5]. Adolescents that experience cognitive decline are at higher risk for mental illness at some point during their disease process [5].

Even though these teenagers have been diagnosed with a significant and life-altering disease, psychiatric issues are often overlooked [1]. When assessing various psychosocial issues that may arise with chronic illness, depression is likely the most common associated psychiatric diagnosis. The statistics vary greatly, but it is thought that between 20-50% of adolescents diagnosed with MS will experience some level of depression [5]. Due to the loss of normal physical function, there is often a grief reaction associated [6]. As socialization is decreased, often due to physical constraints or limitations, peer relationships weaken or dissolve [6]. Anxiety also occurs commonly as a result of the fear of disease progression and the fear of the unknown, specifically with regards to future physical and cognitive functional decline [5]. Other affective disorders, including panic and bipolar disorders, can also arise in these patients [1]. Aggression and hyperactivity have been noted in a small percentage of these teens [5]. Neurologists are often not comfortable with the diagnosis and management of the commonly associated psychiatric issues, so they will often defer to psychiatrists, psychologists, and therapists for assistance in management [4].

The decline in daily functioning is one of the greatest causes for psychosocial issues in the adolescent MS population. 20-50% of these individuals will experience significant fatigue [3], which greatly limits their school attendance [4]. Many of these teens will stop participation in sports due to physical impairment and risk of injury [7], which contributes to social isolation [5]. A large number of these adolescents with suffer from a lack of motivation [7] and it is common to see a decline in school performance and grades [3].

There are many concerning behaviors that can occur due to ineffective coping and poor decision making in adolescents diagnosed with MS, especially in the initial adjustment period. For various reasons, some of these teens will chose to participate in high risk behaviors. Poor medication compliance is a common concern with chronically ill teenagers [4]. Some of these adolescents will act out in school, leading to various disciplinary actions taken by school officials, including suspension [4]. Experimenting with tobacco, alcohol, and illicit drugs may occur and is something that should be monitored closely [4]. Running away from home, promiscuous sexual behavior, and criminal activity are more extreme behaviors that can occur in adolescents with a chronic illness [4]. Self-harm and even suicidal ideations and suicide attempts are very concerning behaviors that should be managed aggressively in these individuals [4].

Dysfunction is not always the end result when adjusting to a chronic disease [4]. Even though adolescence is a difficult time to navigate for a healthy teenager, there are many things that can be done to ensure effective coping during this transition. It is crucial to employ an interdisciplinary approach to caring for these kids [6]. Studies have shown that having a strong support system in place is essential for the best outcomes. In all youth, positive parent-child relationships have been shown to improve resiliency in kids facing major stressors [8]. Maintaining open dialogue within the family regarding the diagnosis of MS is an important way to help adolescents cope emotionally [5]. Parents should be considered protectors and advocates [7]. Teenagers also adapt better to chronic illness if they have a supportive group of peers that are well informed on their disease process [9].

Due to physical and cognitive impairments, school performance can rapidly decline after MS diagnosis [3]. As with all chronically ill students, teens with MS are frequently absent and quickly become behind in their school work. Absenteeism, paired with a decline in cognitive functioning and memory, can create a frustrating and difficult learning environment for these adolescents [3]. Early identification of potential school related issues is important [7]. If needed, the student should be accommodated with favored seating to help with any vision problems or to reduce distractions, decreasing the work load and allowing extra time for assignment completion, and individualized organization or reminders to help with memory loss [4]. Adolescents with MS may benefit greatly from the use of technology to assist with hearing, vision, and writing. Occupation therapy may also be useful in helping with motor and cognitive skills [4]. The best outcomes are noted when school teachers and officials are supportive of the individual needs of these teens and are willing to work with parents and medical providers to ensure that they are getting the services that they need to succeed in school.

Healthcare providers need to be strong advocates for adolescents diagnosed with chronic illnesses like MS. It is important that an interdisciplinary approach is taken [6]. Neurology and primary care providers should work together to meet the basic medical needs, but mental health should not be overlooked. Referrals to psychiatrists, psychologists, and therapists should be a priority upon diagnosis [4]. Even if there are no mental health concerns immediately, it is important for the family to have a resource available if concerns do arise. There are also preventative measures that can be taken to help avoid future issues [4]. Physical, occupational, and speech therapies may be helpful at different stages of the disease process. As with all chronically ill children, health care providers have to remain very involved with the care of the patient and the entire family [4].

CONCLUSION

Multiple sclerosis is a difficult diagnosis for anyone at any age. The adolescent population is extremely vulnerable and must be cared for differently than adults [10]. It is essential that parents, school officials, and medical providers work closely and take a collaborative approach when caring for these teens. There is still room for future research when it comes to the overall psychosocial needs of these individuals. With positive support from all those involved in care, the adolescent can navigate these difficult years in a healthy way.

REFERENCES

[1] Goretti B., Ghezzi A., Portaccio E., Lori S., Zipoli V., Razzolini L. et al. Psychosocial issue in children and adolescents with multiple sclerosis. *Neurol Sci* 2010;31:467-70.

[2] Erikson E. H. *Childhood and Society,* 2nd ed. New York: W. W. Norton; 1963.

[3] Amato M. P. Cognitive and psychosocial issues in pediatric multiple sclerosis: Where we are and where we need to go. *Neuropediatrics* 2012;43:174-5.

[4] MacAllister W. S., Boyd J. R., Holland N. J., Milazzo M. C., Krupp L. B. The psychosocial consequences of pediatric multiple sclerosis. *Neurology* 2007;63: S66-S69.

[5] Till C., Udler E., Ghassemi R., Narayanan S., Arnold D. L., Banwell B. L. Factors associated with emotional and behavioral outcomes in adolescents with multiple sclerosis. *Mult Scler J* 2012;18;1170-80.

[6] Thannhauser J. E. Grief-peer dynamics: Understanding experiences with pediatric multiple sclerosis. *Qual Health Res* 2009;19:766-77.

[7] Boyd J. R., MacMillian. Experiences of children and adolescents living with multiple sclerosis. *J Neurosci Nurs* 2006;37:334-42.

[8] Gribble P. A., Cowen E. L., Wyman P. A., Work W. C., Wannon M. and Raoof A. Parent and child views of parent-child relationship qualities and resilient outcomes among urban children. *J Child Psychol Psychiatry* 1993;34:507-19.

[9] La Greca A., Bearman K. Moore H. Peer relationships of youth with pediatric conditions and health risks: Promoting social support and healthy lifestyles. *J Dev Behav Pediatr* 2002; 23:271-9.
[10] Amato M. P., Goretti B., Ghezzi A., Lori S., Zipoli V., Portaccio E. et al. Cognitive and psychosocial features of childhood and juvenile MS. *Neurology* 2008;70:1891-7.

In: Multiple Sclerosis in Children … ISBN: 978-1-53612-979-3
Editors: H. Omar and J. Chalkley

Chapter 8

PEDIATRIC MULTIPLE SCLEROSIS: EFFECTS ON FAMILY AND FRIENDS

Stephanie Stockburger*, MD and Jennifer Perry, LCSW
Division of Adolescent Medicine and Young Parent Programs, Kentucky Clinic, Department of Pediatrics, Kentucky Children's Hospital, University of Kentucky College of Medicine, Lexington, KY, US

ABSTRACT

Pediatric multiple sclerosis affects not only the individual but also significantly affects family and friends. Roles and relationships may change. Parents or guardians must take on the role of caregiver for a child or adolescent with multiple sclerosis in addition to their parenting and child-rearing duties. A hallmark of multiple sclerosis is relapsing and remitting symptoms. However, some symptoms do not remit and become chronic. An individual may become affected in many ways including sensation, hearing, vision, speech, and movement. As a result, physical, social, and economic effects are an inevitable part of the disease. Good

* Correspondence: Stephanie Stockburger, MD. Department of Pediatrics, Division of Adolescent Medicine. 740 S. Limestone, Lexington, KY 40536. E-mail: sjstoc2@uky.edu.

change over time. Pediatric MS may affect the family and friend relationships in many ways including physically, socially, and economically.

PHYSICAL EFFECTS

Children and adolescents with MS may have relapsing and remitting or chronic physical impairments [2]. Impairments may be present in sensation, vision, hearing, and mobility. Limited mobility may restrict social interactions such as going out with friends and may significantly affect extra-curricular activities such as sports [3]. In the home, special equipment such as a wheelchair, special showers and toilets may be needed if limited mobility is present [3]. Housing that is wheelchair accessible may be needed [3]. In cases of significant immobility, a lift or special bed may be required [3]. An individual with MS may need assistance with personal care such as eating, toileting, and bathing. Motor vehicles may have to be adapted to be wheelchair accessible [3]. The relapsing and remitting nature of MS means that it is important to expect the unexpected. A child or adolescent's mobility status may change over time and it is important for the parent or guardian to be prepared for the possibility of this happening [4].

SOCIAL EFFECTS

The physical effects of MS cause a ripple effect on the social network of the affected child or adolescent and their family and friends [1]. While the individual affected feels the effects of MS firsthand, it is important to remember that those close to them are also affected by the MS. Roles of parents may go from working full-time to working part-time or even staying home to take care of their child [5]. Regardless of the physical impairments of the individual, time off will be needed for medical appointments. In some cases, parents or guardians are administering injections or other treatments to their children or adolescents [4, 5]. Siblings in the household my feel like the individual with MS is getting extra attention and become angry or resentful [5]. Friends of the individual may feel intimidated by the diagnosis and relationships may be stressed [1]. This is particularly significant in adolescence, when the typical developmental stages involve becoming more independent from one's family and closer to one's friends [5]. An adolescent with MS may become frustrated and possibly depressed or anxious if there is a lack of independence and a lack of beginning to start separating from one's family as a result of their chronic disease.

School performance may be affected depending on the level of impairment caused by MS symptoms. School may be missed for doctor's appointments or for physical or occupational therapy. An individual may develop depression or anxiety associated with their diagnosis and may have difficulty focusing in school and may become more despondent from friends. A child or adolescent may also develop MS-related fatigue and lack the energy needed for studying and spending time with friends [1]. Sleep can be affected which can cause further mood disturbance [1, 4].

Finding support for the family and affected child or adolescent is critical. It is important for the child or adolescent to know that other people their age are experiencing similar symptoms and that they are not alone. Encourage the child or adolescent to maintain their friendships. Friends may be intimidated by the diagnosis and simply not understand it. Children often think illnesses are "contagious" and may need developmentally appropriate education about multiple sclerosis to understand what their friend is going through. Children with the diagnosis would benefit from the same education. Schools could aide in acceptance of the diagnosis by providing education about multiple sclerosis or other chronic illnesses and provide factual information as well as how to provide social support for affected children or adolescents. A child or adolescent with MS has a greatly improved quality of life with strong social support from their friends.

It is critically important for caregivers to take time to care for their own health, including their own mental health [4]. It can be difficult for a parent or guardian to adjust to becoming the caregiver of a child or adolescent with MS. Parents and guardians need to feel supported and have their own personal needs met [4]. Many parents and guardians find support through MS support groups either in-person or online [4]. In addition, parents and guardians need to make time to keep their own relationships healthy [4]. A supportive religious community is often helpful [4, 5]. Caregivers should continue to keep up with their own personal health including doctor visits [4]. Families may benefit by reaching out for help with activities such as grocery shopping, doing laundry, and transporting children [4]. It is important to reach out to help prevent caregiver burnout. Caregivers that are experiencing burnout may have difficulty providing effective care due to feeling exhausted and overwhelmed [4].

Economic Effects

Family relationships may be strained by economic factors related to the child or adolescent's MS. The economic strain can be compounded if the parent or guardian has decreased hours at work or decided to stop working in order to provide care thus resulting in decreased household income [4]. Treatments for MS may be costly and may not be covered, or completely covered, by insurance. The economic effect on the family may vary greatly based on the affected individual's insurance. Currently, a main political focus in the United States is on healthcare reform. With the passage of the Affordable Care Act under President Obama's administration in 2010, individuals are allowed to stay on parent's insurance plans until the age of 26. Insurance is currently available to those with "pre-existing conditions." If this aspect of the Affordable Care Act is repealed, older adolescents and young adults with MS will be left with a huge economic burden. They would be considered "uninsurable" due to having a pre-existing condition. This would leave the individual or family to pay out-of-pocket for medical appointments, hospital stays, and treatments. Likely, many individuals with MS would simply go without care instead of incurring significant financial burden. Life-saving treatments may not be attainable and the quality of life for individuals with MS would be lessened very quickly.

In addition to the above-mentioned financial strains, if an individual has difficulty with mobility a number of expensive adjustments may be needed. A single story house may become necessary as well as a wheelchair accessible vehicle [3]. Also in this case, an individual may need assistance with activities of daily living [3]. Services to provide this kind of care can be costly [4]. An individual may also be unable to be left at home unattended due to safety reasons if there is limited mobility [4]. In this case, care would need to be provided to the individual while the caregiver is running errands or working [4].

A child or adolescent with MS may need to take breaks from school during relapses. This may put the individual behind academically [2]. For adolescents in high-school or college this may lead to significant economic burden due to prolonging the time spent in the educational setting. As a result, entry into the workforce may be delayed. Adolescents who have a job may need to ask for time off for medical appointments. A relapse may be frustrating to employers as an individual has no way of knowing how long a relapse will last and if the symptoms will resolve completely.

CONCLUSION

Pediatric multiple sclerosis affects not only the individual but also their family and friends. Restricted social interaction may lead to decreased quality of life for all involved. Open communication and being proactive early on is crucial for maintaining healthy relationships [4]. While some effects of multiple sclerosis may be out of an individual's control, such as debilitating symptoms and adverse consequences of political decisions regarding healthcare coverage, many effects are able to be mitigated. For children and adolescents maintaining contact with friends and social networks is critical. Helping adolescents feel as independent as possible is important for their developmental needs. Parents and guardians functioning as primary caregivers for children and adolescents with MS can reach out to friends, support groups, and religious activities [4]. It is important for caregivers to continue to maintain marriages and relationships [4]. With a strong social support network, children and adolescents with multiple sclerosis can enjoy a remarkably enhanced quality of life despite the difficulties that can accompany their diagnosis.

REFERENCES

[1] Halper, J. The psychosocial effect of multiple sclerosis: the impact of relapses. *J. Neurol. Sci.* 2007; 256:S34-8.

[2] National Multiple Sclerosis Society. *Pediatric MS*. Accessed 2017 Mar 31. URL: http://www.nationalmssociety.org/What-is-MS/Who-Gets-MS/Pediatric-MS.

[3] National Multiple Sclerosis Society. *Mobility and Accessibility*. Accessed 2017 Mar 31. URL: http://www.nationalmssociety.org/Living-Well-With-MS/Mobility-and-Accessibility.

[4] National Multiple Sclerosis Society. *A Guide for Caregivers*. Accessed 2017 Mar 31. URL: http://www.nationalmssociety.org/nationalmssociety/media/msnationalfiles/brochures/brochure-a-guide-for-caregivers.pdf.

[5] National Multiple Sclerosis Society. *Family and Relationships*. Accessed 2017 Mar 31. URL: http://www.nationalmssociety.org/Living-Well-With-MS/Family-and-Relationships.

In: Multiple Sclerosis in Children … ISBN: 978-1-53612-979-3
Editors: H. Omar and J. Chalkley

Chapter 9

The Financial Burden of Pediatric Multiple Sclerosis

Cori Morgan**, APRN, FNP-C

Division of Adolescent Medicine and Young Parent Programs,
Kentucky Clinic, Department of Pediatrics,
Kentucky Children's Hospital,
University of Kentucky College of Medicine,
Lexington, Kentucky, US

Abstract

Pediatric multiple sclerosis (MS) is a chronic and debilitating disease associated with frequent hospitalizations and high health care costs. Although the diagnosis of pediatric MS is a relatively new and rare, steps must be taken in the future to reduce the substantial costs to the United States health care system and families suffering from effects of this disease. Direct and indirect costs related to pediatric MS include hospitalizations, diagnostic testing, drug therapy, missed school, and parental leave from work. Accurate and timely diagnosis, reduction in the cost of treatment, adequate health care coverage, and an understanding of

* Corresponding Author E-mail: cearen2@uky.edu.

the financial burden of MS are important steps in improvement of its monetary impact. A great deal of attention and research is required to address and decrease the financial burden of pediatric MS.

Keywords: multiple sclerosis, pediatric, financial, cost, burden, insurance, DMTs, family, therapy

INTRODUCTION

Multiple sclerosis (MS) is a chronic, unpredictable, cyclic, and debilitating neurologic disease. The central nervous system is made up of neurons that are made of a cell body and an extension of the cell body called the axon which allows the system to transport messages. In MS the immune system damages the central nervous system as it mistakenly attacks the myelin covering neuronal axons which inhibits the body's ability to carry messages correctly [11]. Multiple sclerosis is Greek for "many scars," which refers to the areas of myelin damage known as plaques or lesions that fill in with scar tissue. MS is a multifactorial disease; in that the etiology of it is not completely clear [5]. Autoimmune, environmental, and genetic factors play an important role in its process [5]. MS is extremely variable and its clinical and pathologic process may change frequently. MS is categorized into four subtypes, including clinically isolating syndromes, relapsing-remitting, secondary progressive, and primary progressive. There are approximately 450,000 individuals in the United States living with this disease, and the national incidence rates of adult and pediatric MS have steadily increased over the last half century [15].

Pediatric multiple sclerosis is defined by patients with an onset of the disease before the age of 18. In the pediatric population, MS is diagnosed at approximately 15 years of age. In 97-99% of children diagnosed, relapsing-remitting is the initial form of disease [20]. Although MS is a similar process in adults and children, initial presentation can be vastly different in pediatric patients. Initial features may include cerebellar and brainstem symptoms, encephalopathy, and seizure activity [3]. Common relapse features of pediatric patients include vision loss, sensory disturbances, weakness, balance difficulty, and gait instability [15]. Pediatric MS is rare and only makes up approximately 5% of all MS cases [11]. Since there is such a small incidence of the disease, pediatricians and pediatric neurologists consider several other diagnoses before identifying MS. It wasn't until 2001 that the first diagnostic criterion was created for accurate assessment of the disease which is known as the McDonald Criteria [13]. There have been several revisions of the McDonald criteria since 2001, and the diagnosis continues to remain very challenging for providers today [10].

COST OF NEWLY DIAGNOSED MS

Multiple Sclerosis is associated with significantly high expenses, especially within the first 12 months of diagnosis. The highest cost incurred in pediatric MS is at the onset of the disease process [21]. Cost of services are substantially higher for MS versus healthy patients of inpatient services ($4,110 vs. $836), radiology services ($1,693 vs $259), office visits ($843 vs $310) and therapies ($295 vs $81) [2]. Those with MS are around 3.5 times more likely to be hospitalized, 2 times more likely to be have an emergency department visit, and 2.4 times more likely to have a minimum of one physical, occupational, or speech therapy visits during this time. Overall, medical costs are at least 4.7 times higher for a newly diagnosed MS patient compared to a healthy individual [2].

Since pediatric MS is a rare disease, the search for an accurate diagnosis contributes to family's health care costs. Until the 1990s it was not generally known by medical providers that MS existed in the pediatric population [5]. Subjective symptoms in children are often overlooked and not investigated completely which may delay the identification of MS until adulthood [5]. Time of diagnosis from initial onset of symptoms averages approximately twenty-three months [10]. This delay of diagnosis causes frequent acute and unnecessary visits to general practitioners and contributes to outpatient associated costs [10]. The utilization of pediatric neurology referral, imaging tools, and McDonald Criteria can decrease delay in treatment commencement. Unfortunately there is limited availability to pediatric MS treatment centers in the United States, and families likely have to travel great distances to have their care managed [12].

Imaging studies required for diagnosis and assessment of MS progression are another costly component of MS. Following diagnosis of MS, recommendations suggest that brain MRIs are to be complete every 6 months to monitor disease activity and treatment effectiveness in pediatric patients [3]. In the United States there is much variation in the cost of MRIs. Such imaging studies range from $300 to $3000 based on several factors, such as the type of facility obtaining the scan, quality of the machine, and patient insurance coverage [19].

Cost of Drug Therapy

There are many methods of medication treatment of the varying stages of MS practiced in adults, but a large majority of treatment lacks FDA approval in pediatric patients [5, 6]. Additional research could lead to an increase in patient adherence and more efficient treatment. Approximately 40% of pediatric MS patients suspend medication treatment. This discontinuation of therapy is generally due to intolerance, toxicity, persisting relapses, and nonadherence [11]. Despite a lack of treatment guidelines, pediatric neurologists use adult approved drugs for management [5, 6]. Acute treatment of the disease includes the use of corticosteroids, IVIG, and plasmapheresis [18]. For relapse prevention, immunomodulatory treatments such as injectable interferon-beta 1a or glatiramer and oral agents such as fingolimod, teriflunomide, and dimethyl fumerate may be used [18]. Immunosuppressant drugs are used during refractory periods that include cyclophosphamide, rituximab, and natalizumab for treatment [18].

There has been an exponential increase in cost of all MS drugs over the last few decades that are essential for disease management [8]. The cost of first generation disease-modifying therapies (DMTs) increased from approximately $8,000 to $11,000 annually in the 1990s to an astounding $60,000 per year in current times [8]. The rates of MS drugs are climbing at a speed four to five times higher than typical drug inflation [8]. DMTs in the United States are two to three times the price of DMTs in other industrialized countries [8]. In addition, newer generation disease-modifying drugs can cost up to 60% more than first generation therapies [8].

COST ASSOCIATED WITH INSURANCE COVERAGE

The Affordable Health Care Act (ACA) was signed into law in 2010 to provide medical care to all people across the United States. The ACA requires American citizens to purchase health insurance through their employers or the health insurance exchange and avoid paying a tax penalty for not being insured [7]. The ACA ensures that insurance companies may not cancel or deny family coverage based on pre-existing conditions, provide free preventative care, and allow young adults to stay on their parent's plans until the age of 26 years old. The ACA also bans insurance companies from setting lifetime and yearly maximums, which is crucial in maintaining financial security in Americans with chronic diseases. Although citizens in the United States now have greater access to health insurance, associated costs of co-pays, premiums, and deductibles are expensive for families [7]. In 2014 the median individual deductible was $2500 while the maximum was $6250, and the median drug deductible is $400 and maximum is $2500 [7]. Along with paying high premiums on a monthly basis, deductibles must be met before insurance companies begin paying for treatment. Insurance frequently denies medications required for disease management which is frustrating to individuals and medical providers [8].

Deciding which treatment is necessary for pediatric MS patients is a complex process that requires shared decision making between families and medical providers [8]. Unfortunately, limitations insurance companies place on medication availability can deeply disrupt those shared decisions and may cause harm to the patient [8]. There is no standard health insurance that exists in the United States that guarantees the coverage of any specific medication needed to for an individual. Coverage of immunomodulatory therapies for MS patients varies due to several factors. Medications may be denied or delayed by insurances because of patient's region of residence, predetermined approved medication preference, communication errors between providers and insurance, type of insurance tier coverage purchased, and requirements of prior authorization [6]. Neurologists estimate that a minimum of 1 to 1.5 hours weekly is dedicated to dealing with denied medications of insurances [8]. Oftentimes families are at the mercy of their insurance coverage and state health assistance despite what the most appropriate treatment may be for the individual [7, 17]. Family units with a member suffering from MS are responsible for medication therapies, insurance premiums, and high cost of inpatient and outpatient treatment while attempting to cover daily family expenses [15].

Indirect Costs

Symptoms of MS usually emerge during adolescence which is a critical time for physical, emotional, and mental development. MS may compromise the psychological well-being of the patient as well as family [12]. Adolescent patients may have difficultly discovering the independence that is necessary to development. Associated conditions with MS such as depression and cognitive disability require supplementary treatment such as therapy and additional medication [15, 5]

Sometimes children take a leave of absence from school and are unable to participate in their normal daily activities. At disease onset and throughout the course of MS guardians may take time off or quit their jobs to maintain a flexible schedule for their child's appointments and hospital admissions [12].

Studies suggest that spending any more than 10% of total family income on health care is considered a financial burden on the family [16]. Children with special health care needs (SHCN) are defined as children who need health services beyond what is typically required by children.

Currently, there isn't data specific to total cost burden of families with patients with pediatric MS. Of children with special health care needs, out-of-pocket medical expenditures (excluding insurance premiums) range from $2,669 to 69,906 compared to S676 to $3,181 for families with children without SHCN [16]. In children with SHCN great financial burden is perceived by parents that have lost income due to cutting hours or quitting their jobs. Families perception of burden raises significantly based on the severity of their child's health condition [16].

Parent's inability to work can result in selling assets, obtaining additions loans, draining savings, and filing bankruptcy [16]. It was proposed that in 2009 in the United States 62.1% of all personal bankruptcies are related to medical costs [8]. One of the goals of the ACA was to decrease the cost burden that may lead to bankruptcies in the uninsured and underinsured [6]. Families indisputably experience a high level of financial strain related to high cost associated with MS. There is a great need for these costs be recognized and addressed so that steps may be taken to decrease the heavy emotional and monetary burden these families must endure.

OVERALL COST OF TREATMENT

Although the course of MS is inconsistent, the financial burden that it brings to families and individuals is constant and significant. This variable disease starves families of the treasured consistency that is known to those without chronic illness. Children with general chronic medical conditions make up only approximately 0.4 to 0.7% of all children in the United

States but they account for approximately 15-33% of all pediatric healthcare costs. It is estimated that the cost of pediatric chronic medical conditions is $50 to $110 billion annually [14]. Health care costs specific to patients with MS are estimated to be staggering. Children with general neurologic impairments account for approximately 29% of charges at children's hospitals [4]. When compared to other chronic conditions, adult MS ranks second behind congestive heart failure in direct all-cause medical costs. This places the financial burden of MS above that of diabetes, injuries, stroke, mental illness, and heart disease [1].

Little research has been devoted to the financial impact of pediatric MS on families. It is estimated that the lifetime cost of pediatric-onset MS will greatly exceed the lifetime cost of treatment of adult-onset MS [15]. Pediatric MS costs associated are direct and indirect. Direct costs include includes the direct costs of hospital-based care, outpatient care, medication therapies, diagnostics, and travel. Indirect costs include missed work and employment issues of parents and associated conditions of the disease [15, 5]. It has been reported that families with one disabled member with MS have a 15% lower median income than other families [12]. Determining the specific cost for a family with a pediatric MS patient greatly depends on availability of resources in their area, the type of insurance coverage carried, and severity of the patient's disease [12].

Outpatient visits represent the highest majority of expenditures of pediatric patients accounting for approximately 83% of total annual cost of disease [21]. This varies significantly compared to majority of costs associated with adult treatment. The average total annual cost for an adult MS patient living in the United States in 2013 was approximately $41,000 [15], where the highest direct cost of adult treatment was modification therapy drugs [1]. Children have more relapses in the first two years of MS onset than adults, which correlates to more hospitalizations early in their disease course and a higher cost burden per patient compared to adult cost burden [15]. It is estimated that the cost per pediatric MS admission alone to be $38,000 not including cost of outpatient visits and drugs associated with the disease course [15]. The financial burden of pediatric MS can be as incredibly debilitating as the disease itself.

possibly because of their metabolic clearance of vitamin D being faster than those with normal body weight [8].

Complementary and Alternative Medicine Therapies

In addition to diet, up to 70% of patients with MS have tried complementary and alternative medicine therapies [9]. Dietary supplements commonly used include omega-3, lipoic acid, ginkgo biloba, ginseng, green tea polyphenols, and vitamin D. Of these, the supplements identified as warranting further research were omega-3, lipoic acid and vitamin D [9]. There are several possible mechanisms by which diet may have an effect on MS. Polyunsaturated fatty acids (PUFAs) are involved in biogenesis of multiple inflammatory molecules [1]. Various immune cell populations have receptors for PUFAs, so they can directly act on immune cells and have immunosuppressive effects [1].

Two placebo-controlled clinical trials studied supplementation with omega-3 fatty acids. A population of 312 people with MS was studied for 2 years, taking 10g fish oil daily [10]. They had less disability progression and fewer relapses than those taking the placebo. The difference was not statistically significant, but there was a trend favoring the fish oil (omega-3) group [10]. A more recent pilot study at Oregon Health & Science University School of Medicine in Portland found that patients with secondary progressive MS taking a daily high dose of lipoic acid reduced whole brain atrophy compared against a placebo [11]. Lipoic acid is a naturally occurring antioxidant that is available over the counter. This randomized, double-blind study was done in adults ages 40 to 70 years old. Twenty-seven participants received 1200 mg of lipoic acid every day for 2 years, while the remaining 24 participants received a placebo [11]. The brain volume of each participate was assessed at study baseline using MRI scans. The researchers found that those who took the lipoic acid showed a 68 percent reduction in the rate of whole brain atrophy [11]. Vitamin D

Conclusion

Pediatric MS is a serious illness associated with frequent hospitalizations and growing health care costs. A greater appreciation of the financial impact of pediatric MS on families is needed to understand the true cost associated with pediatric MS. Although pediatric MS is a relatively new and rare, steps must be taken in the future to standardize treatment and reduce costs to the United States health care system and individual families suffering from this debilitating disease. There must be an increased awareness of pediatric MS to general providers to ensure patients are diagnosed in an accurate and timely manner and avoid unnecessary inpatient and outpatient visits. Attempts must be made to reduce the significant cost burden of rising prices of MS drugs. These high costs are damaging to the health care system and the quality of life for families with MS. It is also necessary to make health insurance coverage affordable with lower deductibles and premiums to prevent financial burden on families in the United States. In regard to insurance companies, it is essential that a continuation of coverage to young adults up to 26 years old under their existing family plans as well as a continuation of denying the ability to limit annual or lifetime benefits and denying coverage based on pre-existing conditions. Medical providers need to recognize the burden of pediatric MS and make an effort to ensure patients have resources and support needed to decrease costs for families. A great deal of attention and additional research is required to address and decrease the financial burden of pediatric MS.

References

[1] Adelman G., Rane S, Villa K. The cost burden of multiple sclerosis in the United States: a systematic review of the literature. *J Medical Economics* 2013;16:5.

[2] Asche C., Singer M., Jhaveri M., Chung H., Miller A. All-cause health care utilization and costs associated with newly diagnosed multiple sclerosis in the United States. *J Manag Care Pharm* 2010;16:703-12.

[3] Banwell B., Arnold D., Tillema J., Rocca M., Filippi M., Sormani M. MRI in the evaluation of pediatric multiple sclerosis. *Neurology. 2016; 87. S88-S96.*

[4] Berry J., Poduri A., Bonkowsky J. Trends in resource utilization by children with neurological impairment in the United States inpatient health care system: a repeat cross-sectional study. *PLoS Med* 2012;9.

[5] Chabas D., Green A.J., Waubant E. Pediatric multiple sclerosis. *NeuroRx*. 2006;3:264-75.

[6] Chitnis, T. Pediatric multiple sclerosis: escalation and emerging treatments. *Seminars In Neurology*. 2016;36:148-53.

[7] Esper G.J., Hartung D., Avitzur O. The patient protection and affordable care act and chronic neurological illnesses benefits and challenges. *JAMA Neurol*. 2015;72:739-40.

[8] Hartung D., Bourdette B., Ahmed S., Whitham R. The cost of multiple sclerosis drugs in the US and the pharmaceutical industry: too big to fail? *Neurology* 2015. 84:2185-92.

[9] Himmelstein D.U., Thorne D., Warren E., Woolhandler S. Medical bankruptcy in the United States, 2007: results of a national study. *Am J Med* 2009; 122:741-6.

[10] Hinton D., Kirk S. Paediatric multiple sclerosis: a qualitative study of families' diagnosis experiences. *Archives of Disease in Childhood*. 2015;100:623-9.

[11] Joaquin A.P., Timothy E.L. Pediatric multiple sclerosis: current concepts and consensus definitions. *Autoimmune Diseases*. 2013; 2013 1-12.

[12] Kouzoupis A., Paparrigopoulos T., Soldatos M. Papadimitriou G. The family of the multiple sclerosis patient: A psychosocial perspective. *International Review of Psychiatry*. 2010; 22:83-89.

[13] Krupp L., Tardieu M., Wassmer E. International pediatric multiple sclerosis study group criteria for pediatric multiple sclerosis and

immune-mediated central nervous system demyelinating disorders: revisions to the 2007 definitions. *Multiple Sclerosis Journal.* 2013;19:1261-7.

[14] Kuo, D. Z., Melguizo-Castro, M., Goudie, A., Nick, T. G., Robbins, J. M., & Casey, P. H. Variation in child health care utilization by medical complexity. *Maternal and Child Health Journal* 2015; 19: 40–48.

[15] Lavery A., Banwell B., Liu G., Waldman A.. Hospital admission rates for pediatric multiple sclerosis in the United States using the Pediatric Health Information System (PHIS). *Mult Scler Relat* Disord. 2016;9:5-10.

[16] Lindley, L. Mark, B. Children with special health care needs: impact of health care expenditures on family financial burden. *Journal of Child and Family Studies* 2010 19: 79-89.

[17] Mah J.K., Thannhauser J.E. Management of multiple sclerosis in adolescents – current treatment options and related adherence issues. Adolescent Health, *Medicine and Therapeutics*. 2010;1:31-43.

[18] Marcus J.F., Waubant E.L. Updates on clinically isolated syndrome and diagnostic criteria for multiple sclerosis. *The Neurohospitalist.* 2013;3:65-80.

[19] Sze-jung W., Sylwestrzak G., Shah C., DeVries A. Price transparency for MRIs increased use of less costly providers and triggered provider competition. *Health Affai* 2014;33:1391-8.

[20] Waldman A., Ghezzi A., Bar-Or A., Mikaeloff Y., Tardieu M., Banwell B. Multiple sclerosis in children: an update on clinical diagnosis, therapeutic strategies, and research. *The Lancet Neurology*. 2014;13:936-48.

[21] Wright M.A., Korgenski E.K., Bardsley T., Bonkowsky J.L., Candee M.S. Comprehensive population-based determination of pediatric multiple sclerosis health care costs. *Neurology Neuroimmunology & Neuroinflammation*. 2017;4:314.

In: Multiple Sclerosis in Children … ISBN: 978-1-53612-979-3
Editors: H. Omar and J. Chalkley

Chapter 10

MINDFULNESS AND MULTIPLE SCLEROSIS

Mandakini Sadhir**, *MD
Division of Adolescent Medicine and Young Parent Programs,
Kentucky Clinic, Department of Pediatrics, Kentucky Children's
Hospital, University of Kentucky College of Medicine,
Lexington, Kentucky, US

ABSTRACT

Multiple sclerosis is a chronic, debilitating autoimmune condition with unknown etiology. It can have significant impact on quality of life and overall sense of wellbeing. It can be associated with poor sleep, fatigue, mental health disorders such as anxiety, depression and affect interpersonal relationships. Impact of mindfulness based interventions in mental health conditions, chronic illness as well as multiple sclerosis in adults has been widely studied. Several studies have concluded that mindfulness based intervention can be beneficial in improving quality of life, mental health and physical symptoms such as fatigue in adult patients with multiple sclerosis. Current literature suggest that practice of mindfulness based techniques improve cognitive performance, attention, social skills, academic skills, emotional regulation, self-esteem, anxiety,

* Correspondence: Mandakini Sadhir, MD. Department of Pediatrics, Division of Adolescent Medicine. 740 S. Limestone, Lexington, KY 40536. E-mail: m.sadhir@uky.edu.

stress and fatigue in adolescent population. There is, however, limited evidence about utilizing mindfulness based intervention in adolescents with chronic illness. The chapter describes practice of mindfulness and current research in treating symptoms of multiple sclerosis.

Keywords: mindfulness, multiple sclerosis, meditation, anxiety, depression

INTRODUCTION

Multiple sclerosis (MS) is a chronic immune-mediated demyelinating and inflammatory disease of the central nervous system.[1] The exact etiology of multiple sclerosis is still unknown but autoimmune, genetic, and environmental factors play important role in its development [1, 2]. Pediatric-onset multiple sclerosis represents approximately 2 to 10% of MS patients with onset in adolescence [2]. The disease in children and adolescents almost always presents in the relapsing-remittent form leading to physical and cognitive disability [3, 4] Multiple sclerosis can affect growth, identity development, cognition, social, emotional well- being and engagement with education and employment [5]. Adolescents may experience increased vulnerability as well psychological distress due to unpredictable course and extent of neurological symptoms and physical impairment [5, 6] In a study, children with MS experienced more fatigue, reduced exercise capacity and impaired motor performance as compared to healthy children.[7] Fatigue was found to correlate with health related quality of life (HRQoL) [7] Cognitive impairment may be seen in pediatric MS which can affect attention, processing speed, memory and executive function [8]. In addition to physical, neurologic and cognitive impairment, children and adolescents may suffer from anxiety and depression. Similar to adult population, mood disorders may negatively impact health related quality of life (HRQOL) [9]. Recent studies suggest approximately 30% of children and adolescents with pediatric MS have depression [9, 10]. The treatment of multiple sclerosis thus involves multidisciplinary approach with team of neurologists, psychologists, ophthalmologists, physiotherapists, psychiatrists and pharmacologists.

MINDFULNESS

Over the years, mindfulness based interventions have drawn much attention in management of various chronic medical and mental illnesses [11]. Mindfulness meditation has its origins from ancient Eastern meditation practices and Buddhist traditions [12, 13]. Jon Kabat Zinn described Mindfulness as "Paying attention in a particular way, on purpose, in the present moment and non-judgmentally" [13]. It is considered as a process of doing regular mindful practice to cultivate awareness and acceptance of the present moment in a non-judgmental way [13]. Neuroimaging studies have demonstrated functional and structural changes in regions of brain involved in learning, memory, attention and emotional regulation as result of engaging in regular mindful practice and meditation [12, 14]. Meditative techniques have been shown to increase vagal nerve output which reduces heart rate and breathing rate resulting in increased relaxation response [12, 14]. Meditative practices have also shown to decrease cortisol, improve sleep and seem to have beneficial role in various chronic illnesses [14]. Research has demonstrated their efficacy in a wide range of psychological conditions [15].

One of well-known mindfulness based approach was developed by Jon Kabat Zinn and is known as Mindfulness-based stress reduction (MBSR) and Mindfulness based cognitive therapy (MBCT) [12]. Mindfulness Based Cognitive Therapy (MBCT) is a derivative of MBSR, with a greater emphasis on cognitive techniques, designed for specific mental health conditions such as recurrent depression [12, 14, 15]. This approach has been widely studied and various meta analyses have provided support for utility of MBSR in a wide range of clinical populations and health conditions [15]. Mindfulness based Stress reduction is an eight-week program with each session lasting for 2.5 hrs. The program provides mindfulness training through the practice of meditation and hatha yoga

[12, 13]. In each session, learners are taught mindful techniques and encouraged to engage in sharing of their learning experiences and difficulties to understand elements of stress [13, 15, 17]. During these 8 week sessions, program seeks to strengthen ability to focus on the present moment and accept experiences or thoughts as they arise without trying to control them [17]; explore personal experience and paying attention to its emotional and sensory aspects rather than intellectual description; fully accept personal experience with its positive as well as negative elements including feelings of pleasure, joy, frustration, rage, or uneasiness [13, 17]. The participants develop the ability to actively choose which personal experiences to be lived and what elements to be focused, acted upon or examined [17]. In addition, program teaches the ability to give up all pretense of having direct control over reality [12, 17]. It is thought that MBSR contributes to health and well-being by cultivating non-judgmental awareness and acceptance of one's moment-to-moment experience which can have a positive effect on the adaptation to the disease, reduce the psychological burden and improve quality of life [16]. In addition, it seems to reduce the impact of maladaptive coping strategies and fixed, reflexive behavioral, emotional and cognitive patterns [14-16].

Mindfulness Based Intervention in Multiple Sclerosis

The chronic and debilitating nature of multiple sclerosis affect quality of life in adolescents as well as in adults. In addition, mood disorders are common in adults [18] and adolescents with Multiple sclerosis [9]. Studies have investigated role of mindfulness based intervention such as MBSR in alleviating symptoms and improving quality of life in adults. Current evidence suggests improvement in symptoms such as fatigue, anxiety, depression, perceived stress and cognition when utilizing mindfulness based interventions [19-23]. In a quasi-experimental study, data was collected from adults with multiple sclerosis utilizing Multiple Sclerosis

Quality of Life- 54 (MSQOL-54) and Fatigue severity scale [24]. In the study, participants engaged in eight 2hour sessions of mindfulness based stress reduction and conscious yoga program. Study group was found to have improvement in subscales of quality of life that included physical health, energy, emotional well-being, health distress, health perception, and satisfaction with sexual function as well as overall quality of life and fatigue severity as compared to control group [24]. Grossman et al. in his study demonstrated that mindfulness training seemed to improve fatigue, depression in adults with relapsing-remitting and secondary progressive MS [25]. The study also showed broad feasibility, acceptance as well as satisfaction and adherence with mindfulness training program among adults [25]. In another study, Simpson et al. found evidence of improvement in perceived stress, depression, positive affect, anxiety and self-compassion immediately post mindfulness intervention [26]. At three months' post MBSR while improvements in perceived stress diminished, there was improvement in mindfulness, positive affect, self-compassion, anxiety and prospective memory [26].

A systemic review of three randomized control trial studies with 183 participants showed statistically significant beneficial effects relating to quality of life and mental health (anxiety and depression) and fatigue which were sustained at three and six months follow up [27]. Another meta-analysis of four studies found that mindfulness based intervention showed improvement in fatigue with moderate effect size in the population diagnosed with multiple sclerosis, traumatic brain injury and stroke [28]. Mind body approaches such as mindful meditation also seem to have a role in protecting and improving cognitive and brain reserve in multiple sclerosis [29].

It has been hypothesized that mindfulness based interventions help people with chronic progressive disease to accept daily challenges, teach them to recognize their thoughts and feelings thereby developing acceptance and self-compassion [30]. Group dynamics may also play a fundamental role in the success of the mindfulness interventions. Decentering and self-efficacy appear to be key mechanisms leading to reduced distress [30]. Previous studies have shown that stress plays a significant role in pathogenesis and progression of Multiple sclerosis. Persistent stress can lead to chronic elevation of cortisol and thought to further complicate response to treatment [31]. Meditative practices including mindful meditation have shown to reduce cortisol and may have beneficial role in treatment of multiple sclerosis [31].

MINDFULNESS IN ADOLESCENTS

Adolescence is marked by pubertal growth, psychosocial and cognitive development. Risk taking behaviors [32] and mood disorders [33] are common during this period. Mindfulness based interventions have found to be feasible and acceptable in children and adolescent population [34, 35, 39]. Various studies have shown that mindfulness training and practice in adolescents improves their emotional regulation, attention, cognition, social interaction, sleep and overall sense of well-being [34]. Mindfulness based techniques have been utilized across various settings particularly in schools to address high risk behaviors as well as mental health concerns [36]. Mindfulness based interventions appear to be a promising approach for coping with symptoms related to chronic illness in adolescents. A study demonstrated beneficial effect on depression, quality of life, and acceptance of pain in adolescents with recurrent headaches [38]. Study investigating impact of mindfulness based stress reduction program in adolescents with functional somatic pain syndromes found preliminary evidence of improvement in functional disability, symptom impact and anxiety [41]. Among adolescents and young adults who were cancer survivors, mindfulness based intervention resulted in significant reduction in emotional distress and improvement in quality of life at 3 months of follow-up. In addition, participants had reduced negative attitudes toward self and demonstrated significant improvement in mindfulness skills [42].

Parents of children with chronic medical conditions or disabilities face tremendous difficulties such as child behavioral problems, financial and social barriers in addressing their children health care needs [43]. Studies show that parents undergo psychological stress that impacts their physical, mental health and their relationship with partners, families and children [43]. Addressing parental well-being can be crucial and important part of management of child's health condition. Cognitive behavioral therapy and mindfulness based intervention show promising outcomes among parents. A study found improvement in life satisfaction with regards to spare time, relationship with children and partner when parents utilized mindfulness practice [44]. In another study, caregivers who were mostly mothers with children with special needs and various chronic condition participated in mindfulness based stress reduction (MBSR) sessions. Over the 8-week period, caregivers had overall reduction in mood disturbance and symptoms related to stress [44].

Future Implications

Current literature suggests role of mindfulness based interventions as an adjuvant to traditional treatment of multiple sclerosis in adults. Mindfulness based intervention in adolescents have been utilized to address high risk behaviors as well as mental health concerns. While research is limited, mind-body approach seems to address some aspects of chronic illness in adolescents as well as improving wellbeing of parents and caregivers. Research is needed to investigate impact of mindfulness based intervention in improving symptoms and overall wellbeing of children and adolescents with multiple sclerosis.

References

[1] Chabas D, Green AJ, Waubant E. Pediatric multiple sclerosis. *NeuroRx*. 2006 Apr;3(2):264-75.

[2] Jancic J, Nikolic B et al. Multiple sclerosis in pediatrics: Current concepts and treatment options. *Neurol Ther*. 2016 Dec;5(2):131-43.

[3] Najafi MR, Najafi MA, Nasr Z. Diagnosis and management of multiple sclerosis in children. *Iran J Child Neurol.* 2016 Summer;10(3):13-23.

[4] Chou IJ, Wang HS et al. Pediatric multiple sclerosis: update on diagnostic criteria, imaging, histopathology and treatment choices. *Curr Neurol Neurosci Rep*. 2016 Jul;16(7):68.

[5] MacAllister WS et al. The psychosocial consequences of pediatric multiple sclerosis. *Neurology*. 2007 Apr 17;68(16 Suppl 2):S66-9.

[6] Goretti B, Ghezzi A et al. Psychosocial issue in children and adolescents with multiple sclerosis. *Neurol Sci.* 2010 Aug; 31(4):467-70.

[7] Toussaint-Duyster LC, Wong YYM et al. Fatigue and physical functioning in children with multiple sclerosis and acute disseminated encephalomyelitis. *Mult Scler.* 2017 Apr 1:1352458517706038.

[8] Suppiej A, Cainelli E. Cognitive dysfunction in pediatric multiple sclerosis. *Neuropsychiatr Dis Treat.* 2014;10:1385-92.

[9] Weisbrot DM, Ettinger AB, Gadow KD, et al. Psychiatric comorbidity in pediatric patients with demyelinating disorders. *J Child Neurol.* 2010;25:192-202.

[10] Parrish JB, Weinstock-Guttman B, et al. Fatigue and depression in children with demyelinating disorders. *J Child Neurol*. 2012; 28:713-8.

[11] Gotink RA, Chu P et al. Standardized mindfulness-based interventions in healthcare: an overview of systematic reviews and meta-analyses of RCTs. *PLoS One.* 2015;10(4).

[12] Shonin E, Van Gordon W. The Mechanisms of Mindfulness in the Treatment of Mental Illness and Addiction. *International Journal of Mental Health and Addiction.* 2016;14(5):844-9.

[13] Kabat-Zinn, J. *Full Catastrophe Living: Using the Wisdom of your Body and Mind to Face Stress, Pain, and Illness* Fifteenth Anniversary Edition. 2005. New York, NY: Bantam Dell.

[14] Guendelman S, Medeiros S, Rampes H. Mindfulness and emotion regulation: insights from neurobiological, psychological, and clinical studies. *Front Psychol.* 2017;8:220.

[15] Shapiro SL, Carlson LE. *The art and science of mindfulness: Integrating mindfulness into psychology and the helping professions.* Washington, DC, US: American Psychological Association, 2015; xvii; 194:3-14.

[16] Grossman P, Niemann L, Schmidt S, Walach H. Mindfulness-based stress reduction and health benefits. A meta-analysis. *J Psychosom Res.* 2004 Jul; 57(1):35-43.

[17] Muñoz San José A, Oreja-Guevara C et al. Psychotherapeutic and psychosocial interventions for managing stress in multiple sclerosis: the contribution of mindfulness-based interventions. *Neurologia.* 2016 Mar;31(2):113-20.

[18] Jones KH, Ford DV, Jones PA et al. A large-scale study of anxiety and depression in people with Multiple Sclerosis: a survey via the web portal of the UK MS Register. *PLoS One.* 2012;7(7).

[19] Kolahkaj B, Zargar F. Effect of mindfulness-based stress reduction on anxiety, depression and stress in women with multiple sclerosis. *Nurs Midwifery Stud.* 2015 Dec;4(4).

[20] Krysko KM, O'Connor P. Quality of life, cognition and mood in adults with pediatric multiple sclerosis. *Can J Neurol Sci.* 2016 May;43(3):368-74

[21] Hourihan SJ. Managing fatigue in adults with multiple sclerosis. *Nurs Stand.* 2015 Jun 24; 29(43):51-8.

[22] Bogosian A, Chadwick P, Windgassen S, Norton S, McCrone P, Mosweu I, et al. Distress improves after mindfulness training for progressive MS: A pilot randomised trial. *Mult Scler.* 2015 Aug; 21(9):1184-94.

[23] Senders A, Bourdette D, Hanes D, Yadav V, Shinto L. Perceived stress in multiple sclerosis: the potential role of mindfulness in health and well-being. *J Evid Based Complementary Altern Med.* 2014 Apr; 19(2):104-11.

[24] Nejati S, Rajezi Esfahani S, Rahmani S, Afrookhteh G, Hoveida S. The Effect of Group Mindfulness-based Stress Reduction and Consciousness Yoga Program on Quality of Life and Fatigue Severity in Patients with MS. *J Caring Sci.* 2016 Dec;5(4):325-35.

[25] Grossman P, Kappos L, Gensicke H, D'Souza M, Mohr DC, Penner IK, et al. MS quality of life, depression, and fatigue improve after mindfulness training: a randomized trial. *Neurology.* 2010 Sep 28; 75(13):1141-9.

[26] Simpson R, Mair F, Mercer S. Mindfulness-based stress reduction for people with multiple sclerosis-a feasibility randomized controlled trial. *BMC Neuro.*2017 May16; 17(1):94.

[27] Simpson R, Booth J, Lawrence M, Byrne S, Mair F, Mercer S. Mindfulness based interventions in multiple sclerosis--a systematic review. *BMC Neurol.* 2014 Jan 17; 14:15.

[28] Ulrichsen KM, Kaufmann T, Dørum ES, Kolskår KK, Richard G, Alnæs D, et al. Clinical utility of mindfulness training in the treatment of fatigue after stroke, traumatic brain injury and multiple sclerosis: a systematic literature review and meta-analysis. *Front Psychol.* 2016; 7:912.

[29] Crescentini C, Urgesi C, Fabbro F, Eleopra R. Cognitive and brain reserve for mind-body therapeutic approaches in multiple sclerosis: a review. *Restor Neurol Neurosci.* 2014; 32(5):575-95.

[30] Bogosian A, Hughes A, Norton S, Silber E, Moss-Morris R. Potential treatment mechanisms in a mindfulness-based intervention for people with progressive multiple sclerosis. *Br J Health Psychol.* 2016 Nov;21(4):859-80.

[31] Levin AB, Hadgkiss EJ, Weiland TJ, Jelinek GA. Meditation as an adjunct to the management of multiple sclerosis. *Neurol Res Int.* 2014; 2014:704691.

[32] Kann L, McManus, T, Harris WA et al. Youth Risk Behavior surveillance-2015. *MMWR Surveill Summ* 2016. Jun 10;65(6):1-174.

[33] Michael H. Tang, Elizabeth G. Pinsky. Mood and Affect Disorders. *Peds in Rev*. Feb 2015;36(2):52-61.

[34] Zoogman S, Goldberg, SB, Hoyt WT, Miller, L Mindfulness Interventions with Youth: A Meta-Analysis. *Mindful.* 2015 Apr;6(2):290–302.

[35] Thompson M, Gauntlett-Gilbert J. Mindfulness with children and adolescents: effective clinical application. *Clin Child Psychol Psychiatry.* 2008 Jul;13(3):395-407.

[36] Zenner C, Herrnleben-Kurz S, Walach H. Mindfulness-based interventions in schools-a systematic review and meta-analysis. *Front Psychol.* 2014 Jun 30;5:603.

[37] Ahola Kohut S, Stinson J, Davies-Chalmers C, Ruskin D, van Wyk M. Mindfulness-based interventions in clinical samples of adolescents with chronic illness: a systematic review. *J Altern Complement Med.* 2017 Aug;23(8):581-9.

[38] Hesse T, Holmes LG, Kennedy-Overfelt V, Kerr LM, Giles LL. Mindfulness-Based Intervention for Adolescents with Recurrent Headaches: A Pilot Feasibility Study. *Evid Based Complement Alternat Med.* 2015; 2015:508958.

[39] Waelde LC, Feinstein AB, Bhandari R, Griffin A, Yoon IA, Golianu B. A pilot study of mindfulness meditation for pediatric chronic pain. *Children (Basel).* 2017 Apr 26; 4(5).

[40] Ruskin DA, Gagnon MM, Kohut SA, Stinson JN, Walker KS. A mindfulness program adapted for adolescents with chronic pain: feasibility, acceptability, and initial outcomes. *Clin J Pain.* 2017 Mar 21.

[41] Ali A, Weiss TR, et al. Mindfulness-Based Stress Reduction for Adolescents with Functional Somatic Syndromes: A Pilot Cohort Study. *J Pediatr.* 2017 Apr; 183:184-190.

[42] Van der Gucht K, Takano K, et al. A Mindfulness-Based Intervention for Adolescents and Young Adults After Cancer Treatment: Effects on Quality of Life, Emotional Distress, and Cognitive Vulnerability. *J Adolesc Young Adult Oncol.* 2017 Jun; 6(2):307-317.

[43] Rayan A, Ahmad M. Mindfulness and parenting distress among parents of children with disabilities: A literature review. *Perspect Psychiatr Care.* 2017 Mar 1.

[44] Anclair M, Hjärthag F, Hiltunen AJ. Cognitive behavioural therapy and mindfulness for health-related quality of life: comparing treatments for parents of children with chronic conditions - a pilot feasibility study. *Clin Pract Epidemiol Ment Health.* 2017;13:1-9.

[45] Minor HG, Carlson LE, Mackenzie MJ, Zernicke K, Jones L. Evaluation of a Mindfulness-Based Stress Reduction (MBSR) program for caregivers of children with chronic conditions. *Soc Work Health Care.* 2006; 43(1):91-109.

In: Multiple Sclerosis in Children … ISBN: 978-1-53612-979-3
Editors: H. Omar and J. Chalkley

Chapter 11

MULTIPLE SCLEROSIS AND NUTRITION

Taryn Solomon*[1]*, RDN, LD, CNSC and
Kara Scott*[1,*]*, APRN, DNP, CPNP-PC
[1]Division of Adolescent Medicine and Young Parent Programs,
Kentucky Clinic, Department of Pediatrics,
Kentucky Children's Hospital, University of Kentucky College
of Medicine, Lexington, Kentucky, US

ABSTRACT

Pediatric multiple sclerosis is a complex disease in which the relationship between nutrition and multiple sclerosis (MS) is not well studied. Diet can play a significant role in the body's immune system and central nervous system, therefore, potentially impacting both the onset of MS or the frequency of relapse. Studies have been performed regarding the role of fats, carbohydrates, sugars, salt, vitamin D, omega-3, and lipoic acid in the disease process of MS. Further studies are needed in order to further explore the effects that nutrition has on MS. There are also limited studies specifically related to nutrition, MS, and pediatric patients. Recommendations can be made regarding lifestyle changes and

* Corresponding Author E-mail: kara.scott@uky.edu.

regularly scheduled health maintenance visits in order to optimize patient outcomes and closely monitor nutrition status.

Keywords: multiple sclerosis, pediatric, nutrition, diet

Introduction

The role of diet and nutrition in multiple sclerosis (MS) is largely uncharacterized, particularly as it pertains to pediatric-onset disease. Immunological research has shown that metabolism plays an important role in the function of several immune cells [1]. Bacteria that lives in our gastrointestinal tract plays a big role in our immunity. Gut microbes can act on immune cells and make T-lymphocytes more regulatory by metabolizing diet components into short chain fatty acids [1]. By altering the gut microbial composition, diet can shift the immune system towards a pro- or anti-inflammatory state, possibly even increasing (or decreasing) the risk of some autoimmune diseases [1]. As far as the central nervous system, a change in metabolism may be linked to damage on cellular components such as neurons. This brief chapter discusses how some dietary components can potentially play a role in pediatric multiple sclerosis and disease management.

Iron Intake

A study by Pakpoor, et al. looked at pediatric MS patients from 16 US centers (MS or clinically isolated syndrome onset before age 18) utilizing the food questionnaire Block Kids Food Screener from 2011 – 2016. In unadjusted analyses, there was no difference in intake of fats, proteins, carbohydrates, sugars, fruits or vegetables between the 312 cases and 456 controls [2]. In MS cases, dietary iron intake was lower and they were more likely to consume below recommended guidelines of iron (77.2% of cases vs 62.9% of controls) [2]. This warrants a larger study to establish a relationship between consumption of sufficient iron in pediatric MS cases. No other significant difference in intake of most dietary factors was found [2].

SALT INTAKE

Three studies published by collaborators at Yale, Harvard and MIT/Broad Institute suggest that dietary salt can speed the development of an MS-like disease in mice, and provide new insights on immune system activity involved in MS [3]. Researchers administered salt to human immune cells isolated in lab dishes. They found that higher than normal salt levels dramatically induced activity of immune cells known as T helper 17 (Th17) cells [4]. These immune cells are thought to be important effector cells in MS by producing pro-inflammatory cytokines that disrupt the blood-brain barrier [4]. Another research group explored ways that salt may stimulate the activity of immune cells [5]. They found the protein signaling molecule serum glucocorticoid kinase-1 (SGK1) promotes Th17 cell activity, and both increase when salt concentration increases [5]. This shows that mice fed a high salt diet had more severe disease activity than those fed a normal diet. Particular to pediatrics, a multi-center case-control study was carried out at 14 pediatric MS centers across the country between November 2011 and June 2014 [4]. This study assessed the association between dietary salt intake and pediatric onset of MS risk using data from a large well-characterized set of children. The salt intake was obtained using the Block Kids Food Screener questionnaire. A total of 501 subjects completed the form, met inclusion criteria and remained in the final analysis. This finding did not support a strong association between dietary sodium intake and pediatric onset MS risk, as measured by food questionnaire, BKFS [6]. Although sodium chloride showed no strong correlation to an onset of disease, it is relevant to look at if it can cause a relapse in MS. A frequency in relapse may be helpful in assessing risk factors causing the relapse. A study by Nourbakhsh, et al. utilized a food frequency questionnaire to determine if dietary salt intake is associated with relapse in patients with pediatric-onset MS [7]. In this prospective cohort study carried out between 15 pediatric MS centers in the US, it was found that sodium intake was not associated with time to relapse [7]. Additionally, excess sodium intake had no decrease in time to relapse, as compared with patients with non-excess sodium intake [7]. Further clinical trials are needed to determine whether dietary salt plays a role in human, pediatric multiple sclerosis.

There are currently no dietary recommendations for salt intake in MS patients.

WEIGHT MANAGEMENT

A study by Kavak, K. et al. at the New York State MS Consortium (NYSMSC) in Buffalo, NY studied 184 women with MS between March 2012 and July 2013 [8]. Participants were asked to recall their weight at time of first menstruation and at age 25 as well as height. Body mass index (BMI) was calculated with weight at age 25 then categorized according to class: underweight (< 18.5), adequate (18.5 - 24.9), overweight (25.0 - 29.9), and obese (> 30.0). They were further categorized in two groups, overweight (overweight and obese) and non-overweight (underweight and adequate).

Linear regression analyses were carried out to investigate the association between age at MS onset with weight (at menarche and age 25) and BMI (age 25) [8]. Results showed that participants with an earlier MS onset were heavier both at menarche ($p = 0.042$) and age 25 ($p < 0.001$), and BMI at 25 was also higher in individuals with an earlier onset. Significantly earlier disease onset (26.9 years $\pm$ 9.9) was observed in individuals who were overweight at age 25 compared to those who were not overweight [8].

It is thought that the association between the overweight/obese group and the link to MS is the vitamin D deficiency [8]. Overweight and obese individuals are more likely to be deficient in this fat soluble vitamin,

supplementation and its effects on multiple sclerosis are discussed in another chapter.

CONCLUSION

Despite limitations, food frequency questionnaires completed shortly after disease onset to evaluate the association of various nutrients with MS risk is probably the best attempt at deciphering associations between diet and MS risk. Monitoring weight trends throughout adolescence and childhood will also help establish trends between disease prevalence and body habitus. As of now, we can conclude maintaining a healthy weight in early childhood may be the best preventative measure against early onset MS. Following a healthy lifestyle with physical activity and a diet low in processed foods, refined carbohydrates, saturated fats and higher in omega 3, fiber, fruits, vegetables, whole grains and legumes is also beneficial for lowering risk of heart disease, diabetes, and certain cancers. Vitamin D levels should be checked to determine a need for supplementation if a deficiency exists. Considering the high risk of malnutrition in MS patients, registered dietitians should review the signs and symptoms obtained in a nutritional assessment and diagnosed accordingly. Focusing on other nutritional parameters such as constipation, dysphagia, appetite, food security and food safety will be critical. Registered dietitians can be an important part of a patient's care by observing disease progression and monitoring the ability to consume sufficient calories and protein with or without assistance. Nutritional status will ultimately depend on adequate, safe oral intake and consistently meeting dietary needs.

REFERENCES

[1] Bhargava, Pavan. *Diet and multiple sclerosis.* National Multiple Sclerosis Society 2015. Accessed 2017 July 12. URL:

http://www.nationalmssociety.org/NationalMSSociety/media/MSNationalFiles/Documents/Diet-and-Multiple-Sclerosis-Bhargava-06-26-15.pdf.

[2] Pakpoor, J., Seminatore, B., Graves, J. S., Schreiner, T., Waldman, A. T., Lotze, T. E., Belman, A., et al. Dietary factors and pediatric multiple sclerosis: a case-control study. *Multiple Sclerosis Journal,* 2016; 22(1): 73-4.

[3] National Multiple Sclerosis Society [Internet]. *Supported Studies Point to Possibility That Dietary Salt May Stimulate Activity of Key Immune Cells Involved in MS Attacks.* http:// www.nationalmssociety.org/About-the-Society/News/National-MS-Society-Supported-Studies-Point-to-Pos. Accessed July 12 2017.

[4] Kleinewietfeld, M., Manzel, A., Titze, J., Kvakan, H., Yosef, N., Linker, R. A., et al. Sodium Chloride drives autoimmune disease by the induction of pathogenic TH17 cells. *Nature International Weekly Journal of Science*, 2013; 496(7446):518-22.

[5] Yosef, N., Shalek, A. K., Gaublomme, J. T., Jin, H., Lee, Y., Awasthi, A., et al. Dynamic regulatory network controlling TH17 cell differentiation. *Nature International Weekly Journal of Science*, 2013; 496(7446):461-8.

[6] McDonald, J., Graves, J., Waldman, A., Lotze, T., Schreiner, T., Belman, A., et al. A case-control study of dietary salt intake in pediatric-onset multiple sclerosis. *Multiple Sclerosis and Related Disorders,* 2016; 6:87-92.

[7] Nourbakhsh, B., Graves, J., Casper, T. C., Lulu, S., Waldman, A., Belman, A., et al. Dietary salt intake and time to relapse in paediatric multiple sclerosis. *Jour. Neuro Neurosurg. Psychiatry*, 2016; 87: 1350-3.

[8] Kavak, K. S., Teter, B. E., Hagemeier, J., Zakalik, K., Weinstock-Guttman, B., et al. Higher weight in adolescence and young adulthood is associated with an earlier age at multiple sclerosis onset. *Multiple Sclerosis Journal*, 2015; 21(7): 858-65.

[9] Cunningham, E. Are there evidence based dietary interventions for multiple sclerosis? *Journal of the Academy of Nutrition and Dietetics,* 2013; 113(7): 1004.

[10] National Multiple Sclerosis Society [Internet]. *The Omega-3 Factor.* http://www.nationalmssociety.org/Living-Well-With-MS/Diet-Exercise-Healthy-Behaviors/Diet-Nutrition/Omega-3. Accessed July 12 2017.

[11] Spain, R., Powers, K., Murchison, C., Heriza, E., Winges, K., Yadav, V., et al. Lipoic Acid in Secondary Progressive MS. *Neurology Neuroimmunology and Neuroinflammation,* 2017; 4(5).

In: Multiple Sclerosis in Children … ISBN: 978-1-53612-979-3
Editors: H. Omar and J. Chalkley

Chapter 12

VITAMIN D AND MULTIPLE SCLEROSIS

Victor Kieu**, *MD and Nikki Thaker
Department of Pediatrics, Division of Adolescent Medicine,
University of Kentucky, Lexington, KY, US

ABSTRACT

Multiple sclerosis is a relapsing and remitting autoimmune disease that is often more debilitating, when found in children, than when it occurs in adulthood. Though the exact etiology of MS is unknown, it is well understood that the disease process involves a complex interaction between genetic and environmental factors, of which Vitamin D level, a modifiable environmental factor, has shown a direct correlation with the progression and development of MS risk. In fact, large cohort studies, epidemiology studies, and murine models have shown that a high vitamin D level is most beneficial in MS due to its immunomodulatory effects on T cells specific to the autoimmune process. This new found data has added much promise to the treatment of MS because although one cannot change their own genetic predisposition to the disease, vitamin D level can and should be therapeutically modified for optimal management.

* Correspondence: Victor HT Kieu, MD. University of Kentucky College of Medicine, Kentucky Children's Hospital, Department of Pediatrics. 800 Rose Street, MN 472, Lexington, KY 40536. E-mail: victor.kieu@uky.edu victor.kieu@uky.edu.

Keywords: multiple sclerosis, progression, development, environmental factors, vitamin D, immunomodulatory effects

INTRODUCTION

Multiple Sclerosis (MS) is the most common chronic, immune-mediated, inflammatory, demyelinating disease of the central nervous system. It is not only a physically and psychosocially debilitating disease, but it is also a progressive disease that is not as commonly found in children and adolescents as it is in adults. However, when it does manifest in these younger age demographics, there is increasing evidence that suggests that though the disease process is often slower to manifest in children, that the ongoing insult from such a young age eventually leads to more significant disability long term [1]. As a disease, the etiology is not well understood. It is generally accepted that MS is as a multifactorial disease arising from complex interactions between genetic susceptibility and environmental factors, of which a few are potentially modifiable [2]. Vitamin D deficiency, which has attracted increased attention in the last decade or so is one of those modifiable factors because of its immunomodulatory effects. To date, the best demonstration of the immunomodulatory role of Vitamin D, especially in MS risk, has been shown in mice. In fact, *In vivo*, the induction of $1,25(OH)_2D$ treatments in mice demonstrated inhibition of IL-17 and IFN-γ (inflammatory markers), induction of IL-10 and T reg cells (inflammatory suppressors), and suppression of Th1/Th17 cells (inflammatory regulators), thereby impeding the development and progression of experimental autoimmune encephalomyelitis, the murine model of multiple sclerosis [8].

VITAMIN D: PRODUCTION AND BIOLOGICAL EFFECTS

Vitamin D is a fat soluble vitamin that has 2 main forms, ergocalciferol (vitamin D2), which is plant based, and cholecalciferol (vitamin D3), which is animal based and is the most bioactive form. Though diet through fatty fish and fortified foods do provide some source of vitamin D, the main source for human vitamin D intake is skin exposure to sunlight. In the skin, 7-dehydrocholesterol is photolyzed by ultraviolet radiation from the sun and converted to pre-vitamin D3, which is isomerized to vitamin D3. The vitamin D binding protein then transports vitamin D3 through the blood to the liver where it gets hydroxylated to 25-hydroxyvitamin D3 (25(OH)D3). 25-hydroxyvitamin D3 is further hydroxylated at the kidney to 1,25-dihydroxyvitamin D3 (1,25(OH)2D3), calcitriol, which is the most bioactive vitamin D metabolite [3].

The active vitamin D metabolite calcitriol mediates its biological effects by binding to the vitamin D receptor, which is principally located in the nuclei of target cells [4]. One of the most important roles of vitamin D is to maintain skeletal calcium balance by promoting calcium absorption in the intestines, stimulating bone resorption by increasing osteoclast number, maintaining calcium and phosphate levels for bone formation, and permitting proper functioning of parathyroid hormone to main serum calcium levels [5]. However, vitamin D receptor expression has also been reported in most immune cells, including white blood cells such as monocytes and activated T and B cells, as well as in CNS tissue [4]. In fact, in vitro studies have shown that the addition of 1,25-dihydroxyvitamin D3 to antigen-presenting cells inhibits the surface expression of major histocompatibility complex II-complexed antigens, and of costimulatory molecules, leading to reduced T cell stimulatory capacity. Additionally, 1,25-dihydroxyvitamin D3 directly exerts its immunomodulatory effects on T lymphocytes by inhibiting the production of Type 1 helper T cell cytokines, considered to be the key mediators in graft rejection and autoimmune diseases, and stimulating the production of Type 2 helper T cell cytokines, which have immunoregulatory functions [6]. Furthermore, 1,25-dihydroxyvitamin D3 inhibits T cell and B cell proliferation, blocks B cell differentiation and immunoglobulin secretion, and affects T cell maturation, inducing a shift away from the inflammatory T-helper 17 cells phenotype. All of these immunomodulatory effects of

1,25-dihydroxyvitamin D3 can lead to the protection of target tissue in autoimmune diseases and transplantation [7].

Vitamin D Deficiency and MS: Environmental Exposure vs. Genetic Predisposition

Several epidemiology studies have linked both environmental exposure and genetic predisposition to the effects of Vitamin D levels in lowering the risk towards MS development and/or progression. The most well established phenomenon is the effect of latitude and sunlight exposure on MS risk. This phenomenon highlighted the incidence of MS as being the lowest at the equator and increasing in frequency with distance from the equator. Given the gradations of ultraviolent radiation (UV), only the subtropical and tropical regions, those regions closest to the equator, provide enough UV exposure to produce adequate amounts of vitamin D to fulfill bodily demands. It has been shown in certain studies that MS risk is highest in areas of large portions of the northern and southern hemispheres, away from the equator, with inadequate solar exposure, implicating a negative correlation between MS risk and vitamin D deficiency [10]. In conjunction, other studies have shown that people who have migrated from a high latitude region, with high MS prevalence, to a sunnier region, with lower MS prevalence, were less likely to develop progression towards MS. In addition, adults who spent more time outdoors during childhood had significantly lower risk for MS, indicating yet another association between vitamin D exposure and MS risk [9]. Not to mention, proper Vitamin D supplementation during the first part of life, as early as pregnancy to the end of adolescence has been shown to play a role in decreasing MS risk as well [10]. Furthermore, in a large cohort study, with more than 35,000 mothers and 199 MS cases, daughters of mothers with higher dietary vitamin D intake during pregnancy and higher predicted serum 25(OH)D levels had a 40% lower risk of MS than those whose mothers were in the lowest quintiles [11]. Lastly, in a study involving young white American soldiers, a 41% decrease in MS risk was observed for every 50-nmol/L increase in 25-hydroxyvitamin D [12].

Though various studies have shown a causal relationship between MS risk and Vitamin D deficiency, environmental exposure alone does not implicate an individual to be vitamin D deficient, therefore more prone to progression towards MS. One of the largest cross-sectional studies comparing 339 African Americans with MS vs. 342 African American controls found that not only were 25-hydroxyvitamin D levels lower in African Americans with MS than in the control, but Greater European genetic ancestry was positively correlated with vitamin D status [13]. Thus, it can be concluded that genetic abnormalities of Vitamin D metabolism may also contribute to MS risk, and further fortifies the role of Vitamin D levels in MS risk. Specifically, gene CYP27B1, which encodes 1a-hydroxylase, an enzyme that controls calcitriol synthesis, and genetic abnormalities of the CYP24A1 gene, which encodes the enzyme responsible for initiating calcitriol degradation, have both been associated with MS risk [10]. More recently, single nucleotide polymorphisms (SNPs) associated with 25-hydroxyvitamin D (25OHD) levels have been identified in one of the largest studies to date (n = 33,996), and using Mendelian randomization (MR), researchers showed that genetically lowered vitamin D level influences the risk of MS [14].

ROLE OF VITAMIN D LEVELS IN MS MANAGEMENT

The extensive evidence presented thus far implicates the role of Vitamin D in MS risk, but the exact amount of Vitamin D needed for prevention of relapses and treatment needs to be further studied. For most people, the target 25-OH-D range, derived from multiple metabolic and bone clinical data, is around 30–60 ng/mL or 75–150 nmol/L [10]. Most people with MS present with Vitamin D levels below this range. In a recent study, among 110 subjects, the mean unadjusted 25-hydroxyvitamin D(3) level was 22 +/- 9 ng/ml. Every 10 ng/ml increase in the adjusted 25-

hydroxyvitamin D(3) level was associated with a 34% decrease in the rate of subsequent relapses [15]. Similar results were found in studies conducted in Australia, and Denmark.

While the literature is mixed, Vitamin D may not only play a role in decreasing relapses of MS, but also in long term MS activity and progression. In a randomized trial (n = 334) originally designed to evaluate the impact of early vs delayed interferon beta-1b treatment in patients with MS, serum 25(OH)D concentrations were measured at baseline and at 6, 12, and 24 months. Patients were then followed up for 5 years clinically and by magnetic resonance imaging. Researchers found that higher 25(OH)D levels predicted reduced MS activity and a slower rate of progression. A 50-nmol/L (20-ng/mL) increment in average serum 25(OH)D levels within the first 12 months predicted a 57% lower rate of new active lesions ($P < .001$) on MRI, a 57% lower relapse rate ($P = .03$), a 25% lower yearly increase in T2 lesion volume ($P < .001$), and 0.41% lower yearly loss in brain volume ($P = .07$) from months 12 to 60. In addition, values greater than or equal to 50 nmol/L at up to 12 months predicted lower disability during the subsequent 4 years [16]. While more research is needed to substantiate these findings, preliminary research has laid the groundwork that Vitamin D levels should be monitored and corrected in populations with MS.

CONCLUSION

Multiple Sclerosis is a chronic disease that affects the whole body by directly insulting the myelin sheaths, the protective covering of the tracks of the CNS, causing symptoms such as vision, movement, and sensory disturbances. Until recently, studies regarding modifiable environmental factors, though known, have not gained much traction. In particular, the relationship between Vitamin D levels in MS. Vitamin D is a fat soluble vitamin that is found not only in certain foods, but made by direct sunlight exposure on the skin. It is responsible for calcium homeostasis, but has vast immunoregulatory characteristics. It inhibits the inflammatory characteristics of T1 and T17 helper cells (key mediators in autoimmune diseases), while upregulating inflammatory protective cells such as T2 helper cells. Multiple studies have shown a direct implication on progression and development of MS risk due to Vitamin D levels. In fact, most people with MS present with low Vitamin D levels; a relationship that cannot be ignored. Although studies have varied on the amount of Vitamin D levels needed for symptom protection, it seems as though a level of around 30–60 ng/mL or 75–150 nmol/L is beneficial as an adjunct therapy for the treatment of MS [10].

REFERENCES

[1] National Multiple Sclerosis Society. *Pediatrics MS*; Accessed 2017 June. URL: http://www.nationalmssociety.org/What-is-MS/Who-Gets-MS/Pediatric-MS.

[2] Correale J, Farez MF, Gaitan MI. Environmental factors influencing multiple sclerosis in Latin America. *Mult Scler J Exp Transl Clin* 2017 Apr-June; 3(2).

[3] Alharbi FM. Update in vitamin D and multiple sclerosis. *Neurosciences (Riyadh)* 2015 Oct;20(4):329-35.

[4] Provvedini DM, Tsoukas CD, Deftos LJ, Manolagas SC. 1,25-dihydroxyvitamin D3 receptors in human leukocytes. *Science.* 1983, 221:1181-3.

[5] Bell TD, Demay MB, Burnett-Bowie SA. The biology and pathology of vitamin D control in bone. *Journal of Cellular Biochemistry.* 111(1):7-13.

[6] Van Etten E, Mathieu C. Immunoregulation by 1,25-dihydroxyvitamin D3: basic concepts. *J Steroid Biochem Mol Biol.* 2005;97:93–101.

[7] Aranow C. Vitamin D and the immune system. *J Investig Med.* 2011;59:881-6.

[8] Correale J, Asrraelit M, Gaitán M. Immunomodulatory aspects of vitamin D in multiple sclerosis. *Brain,* 132 (2009), pp. 1146-60.

[9] Forrest KY, Stuhldreher WL. Prevalence and correlates of vitamin D deficiency in US adults. *Nutr Res*. 2011 Jan;31(1):48-54.

[10] Pierrot-Deseilligny C, Souberbielle JC. Vitamin D and multiple sclerosis: An update. *Mult Scler Relat Disord* 2017 May;14:35-45.

[11] Mirzaei F, Michels KB, Munger K, O'Reilly E, Chitnis T, Forman MR, et al. Gestational vitamin D and the risk of multiple sclerosis in offspring. *Ann. Neurol.*, 70 (2011), pp. 30-40.

[12] KL Munger, LI Levin, BW Hollis, NS, Howard, A. Ascherio. Serum 25-hydroxyvitamin D levels and risk of multiple sclerosis. *JAMA*, 296 (2006), pp. 2832-8.

[13] Gelfand, JM, et al. "Vitamin D in African Americans with Multiple Sclerosis." *Neurology* 76. 21 (2011): 1824–1830. PMC. Web. 16 July 2017.

[14] Vitamin D and Risk of Multiple Sclerosis: A Mendelian Randomization Study. Mokry LE et al. *PLoS Med.* (2015).

[15] Mowry EM, Krupp LB, Milazzi M, Chabas D, Strober JB, Belman AL, et al. Vitamin D status is associated with relapse rate in pediatric-onset MS *Ann. Neurol.*, 67 (2010), pp. 618-24.

[16] Ascherio A, Munger KL, White R, Köchert K, Simon KC, Polman CH, et al. Vitamin D as an Early Predictor of Multiple Sclerosis Activity and Progression. *JAMA Neurol*. 2014;71(3):306-14.

In: Multiple Sclerosis in Children … ISBN: 978-1-53612-979-3
Editors: H. Omar and J. Chalkley

Chapter 13

THE FUTURE OF PEDIATRIC MULTIPLE SCLEROSIS

Joshua Chalkley*, DO, MS
Department of Neurology, Neuroimmunology/MS Division,
University of Kentucky, Lexington, KY, US

ABSTRACT

Major strides have been made over the last two decades in terms of understanding, identification, and subsequent treatment of multiple sclerosis. Despite our increased understanding of the disease there remain many challenges. These challenges are especially poignant in pediatric MS which provides a different set of challenges in treating this population. Although there remain challenges in treatment hopefully in the future more patients will live in a disease free state or with significant reduction is disease activity. Significant strides have been made in regards to the understanding of pediatric MS and the first clinical trials are starting to look at treatment effects in these populations. This chapter will briefly review some of the emerging imaging techniques and

* Correspondence: Joshua Chalkley DO, MS. Assistant Professor of Neurology, Neuroimmunology/MS Division. University of Kentucky. 740 South Limestone, Lexington, KY. E-mail: Josh.Chalkley@uky.edu.

concepts which will likely be implemented in the future treatment of pediatric MS.

Keywords: multiple sclerosis, pediatric multiple sclerosis, emerging concepts, future of pediatric MS

Introduction

We are in the midst of a revolution in terms of our understanding, and subsequent treatment of multiple sclerosis over the last two decades. Pediatric multiple sclerosis was initially thought to be vanishingly rare, although uncommon pediatric MS is recognized disease with a steadily growing body of literature. Although the pediatric literature has lagged behind its adult counterparts, significant strides are being made in the field of pediatric MS [1]. Despite this improved understanding, many questions remain. The pathogenesis of multiple sclerosis remains elusive. The etiology of pediatric multiple sclerosis is thought to be similar to that in adults especially in those patients who present in adolescence. However, there is some debate whether prepubertal multiple sclerosis may represent a different pathogenesis. To date there is still no biomarkers for multiple sclerosis either for the diagnosis of the disease, or for subsequent monitoring of the disease. The advent of MR imaging is extremely helpful in the monitoring of inflammatory disease. However, her current monitoring techniques have limitations. We need better clinical tools to monitor the evolution of multiple sclerosis beyond inflammation. We will need new tools to follow patients over the course of their disease [2].

The understanding in treatment of progressive multiple sclerosis remains one of the major challenges in the field. Progressive multiple sclerosis is essentially unheard of in the pediatric population but pediatric patients are at risk for developing secondary progressive MS later in the disease course. Although treatments for progressive MS are emerging this remains a major area of need. At the present time we have no way of healing damaged neuronal tissue. Optimally effective treatment will be able to provide protection from neurologic worsening, and to restore functioning.

There is a substantial body of literature in regards to disease modifying therapy in adult populations, but very little in the way of trial data in pediatrics. Pediatric clinical trials are underway and will hopefully provide guidance in the optimal therapy in our pediatric patients [3].

Measure such as magnetization transfer ratio (MTR) and MRI spectroscopy may be better able to characterize tissue injury over standard MRI. These more sensitive imaging techniques can image cortical and subcortical structures prone to injury in multiple sclerosis which are missed on standard MIR imaging. The realization that multiple sclerosis does effects cortical tissue as well as the subcortical structures was recently recognized, and this offers new direction in how to monitor these structures. Diffusion tensor imaging is another emerging technique which is more sensitive to measuring white matter tracts which may be beneficial in long term monitoring of MS [4].

Ocular coherence tomography (OCT) is a new tool in measuring the damage after optic neuritis, and can demonstrate subclinical change in the optic nerve. Newer generation OCT machines with spectral domain can show reduction in retinal nerve fiber layer. This will provide another way of monitoring degeneration in a quick noninvasive fashion.

In clinic most patients are followed with standard neurological exams, but for the most part these are not quantitated. The timed 25-foot walk, 6-minute walk, 9-hole peg test and "up and go" test all provide measurable scales which can be monitored over time. In the future these are likely to be integrated into standard MS practice to monitor for progression over time. Depression, cognitive function [3].

A growing number of patients with multiple sclerosis are living in a disease free or reduced disease state. The term disease Free State is likely a misnomer and patients may have disease activity which our standard monitoring techniques miss. The proportion of patients living in a disease free state will likely become a new benchmark. Multiple sclerosis is a lifelong disease and patients need monitoring over a significant amount of time to gauge the effect of our current interventions. Several longitudinal studies such as the CLIMB study in Boston are monitoring a large number of patients over decades to assess the efficacy of our current interventions. The concept of induction therapy is gaining some momentum over the last half decade. The concept of permanently changing the immune system from the outset of disease may provide long term benefit and prevent future disability. New treatments such as stem cell transplantation, induction chemotherapy, and emerging treatments for progressive disease are all on the horizon. Higher efficacy may come with a cost, as exemplified by our experience with PML and the development of secondary immune conditions. In the future we will need more sophisticated risk stratification procedures in hopes of selecting the right therapy technique to the patient. There has been some success with risk stratification as exemplified by the risk mitigation with natalizumab associated PML, but these personalized approach is still in its infancy, especially in regards to pediatric patients.

Traditionally neurologist confined themselves to the diagnosis and treatment of MS alone. Given the increasing complexity of MS care this in itself can be a daunting task. There is an emerging trend in medicine, and subsequently neurology to treat the whole person. Over the last decade we have come to recognize how comorbid conditions such as; smoking, obesity, depression negatively influence disease course. Issues like depression, sleep disorders, sexual function, urinary issues and pain are not just common in MS, but major impacts on overall quality of life. In pediatrics academic performance may be the major area affected by their disease, and neurologist traditionally have limited roles in educational experience. The neurologist alone cannot meet all the needs of this complex population. A team approach, were multiple health care providers with different skill sets and expertise are needed to care for the whole patient. The concept of wellness including cognitive behavior therapies, occupational therapy and physical therapy are all needed to provide the best care for our patients.

The ultimate goal for any disease is a cure. Hopefully this will become a reality in the future, but complete resolution of the disease remains elusive. It is clear patients are increasingly living in a reduced disease state, which will hopefully lead to decreased disability over time.

Over the last decade the concept of personalized medicine has emerged were the individual's unique personality, genetic makeup, physiology, disease state, and personal preferences are taken into account when selecting the most appropriate therapeutic option. This is probably best illustrated in oncology when specific hormonal and genetic factors are routinely tested to select therapy. The field of neurology and specifically multiple sclerosis is moving in this direction although there still remain major gaps in the understanding of MS. In the future hopefully we will be able to better identify those patients who will need more aggressive treatment possibly through the aid of a biomarkers or functional imaging would be matched to appropriate therapy. Repair of the nervous systems remains a goal with all neurological disease to help restore normative function. Although, these goals remain out of reach in current clinical practice there is a significant study in the field of pediatric MS. There are multiple prospective clinical trials ongoing which will be the first of their kind in pediatric demyelinating disease. All the oral medications along with Ocrelizumab are currently being studied in a systematic way in children. There is renewed focus on pediatric disease states which will hopefully lead to a better understanding and subsequent treatment of pediatric MS.

REFERENCES

[1] Joaquin, P., Lotze, T. Pediatric Multiple Sclerosis: Current Concepts and Consensus Definitions. *Autoimmune Diseases* 2013; 12.

[2] Rae-Grant, A., Fox, R., Bethoux, F. *Multiple Sclerosis and related disorders clinical guide to diagnosis, medical management, and rehabilitation.* New York: Demos medical, 2013.

[3] Chitnis, T., Ghezzi, A., Bajer-Kornek, B. Pediatric multiple sclerosis escalation and emerging treatments. *Neurology* 2016; 87:103-9.

[4] Filippi, M., Rocca, M. A., De Stefano, N. Magnetic resonance techniques in multiple sclerosis: The present and the future. *Arch. Neurol.* 2011; 68: 1514-20.

SECTION TWO: ACKNOWLEDGMENTS

Chapter 14

ACKNOWLEDGMENTS

I take this opportunity to express my gratitude to my assistant, Laura Whitehouse for her tireless work in helping finalize this book and to Taryn Solomon, who also helped with formatting and finalizing the book.

Hatim Omar, MD
Editor

Chapter 15

ABOUT THE EDITORS

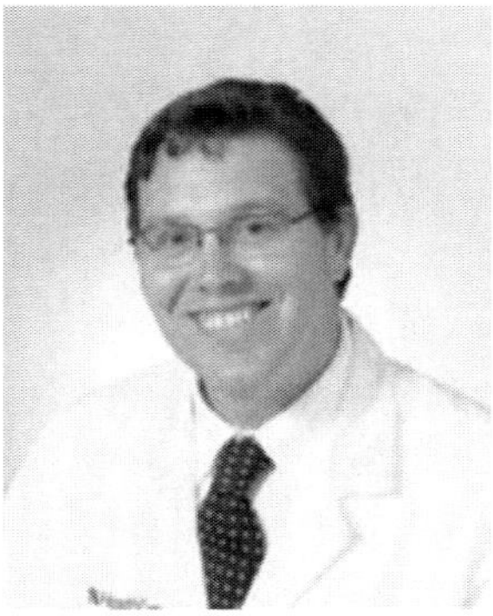

Joshua Chalkley, DO, MS, Assistant Professor of Neurology. He completed his BA in psychology from Asbury University. He went on to obtain additional training in psychology with a master in clinical psychology from Eastern Kentucky University. He completed medical school at Nova Southeastern University and his residency in neurology at the University of Kentucky. He then completed fellowship in neuroimmunology and multiple sclerosis at Brigham and Women's Hospital/Harvard Medical School. Dr. Chalkley is a national MS society clinical fellow recipient. He is an Assistant Professor of Neurology at the University of Kentucky and the director of the University of Kentucky MS

Center. Dr. Chalkley is actively involved in all aspects of multiple sclerosis including direct clinical care, ongoing research and education. E-mail: josh.chalkley@uky.edu

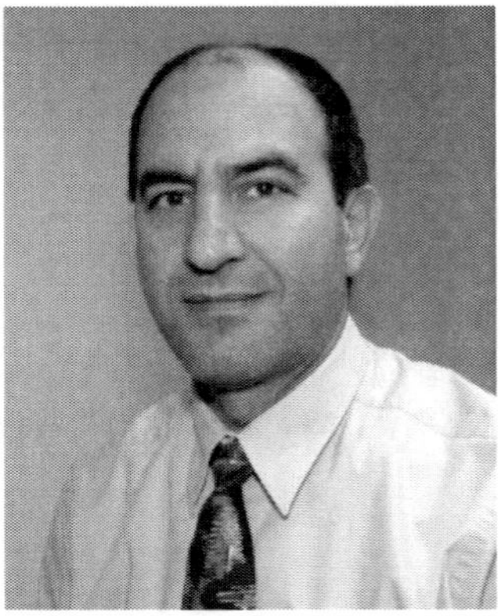

Hatim Omar, MD, FAAP, Professor of Pediatrics and Obstetrics and Gynecology; Professor of Family Studies; and Chief of the Division of Adolescent Medicine, Department of Pediatrics, University of Kentucky, Lexington. He is the holder of the Children's Miracle Network Endowed Chair in Pediatrics. Dr. Omar has completed residency training in obstetrics and gynecology as well as pediatrics. He has also completed fellowships in vascular physiology and adolescent medicine. He is the recipient of the Commonwealth of Kentucky Governor's Award for community service and volunteerism in 2000, Kentucky Teen Pregnancy Coalition Award for outstanding service 2002, Awards for suicide prevention from the Ohio Valley Society for Adolescent Medicine and Kentucky Pediatric Society in 2005 and 2007, Sexual Abuse Awareness Month Award for his work with sexual abuse victims from the Kentucky Association of Sexual Assault Professionals in 2007, Special Achievement Award from the American Academy of Pediatrics 2007 and the Founders of Adolescent Medicine Award from the AAP in 2007. He is well known internationally with numerous publications in child health, public health, pediatrics, adolescent medicine, pediatric and adolescent gynecology. E-mail: haomar2@uky.edu

Chapter 16

LIST OF CONTRIBUTORS

Ana C. Albuja, MD
Chief Resident, J401 Kentucky Clinic, Division of Child Neurology, Department of Neurology, University of Kentucky College of Medicine, Lexington, Kentucky 40536 United States. Email: ana.albuja@uky.edu

Joshua Chalkley, DO MS
Assistant Professor of Neurology, J401 Kentucky Clinic, Neuroimmunology MS Division, Department of Neurology, University of Kentucky College of Medicine, Lexington, Kentucky 40536 United States. Email: josh.chalkley@uky.edu

Kimberly S. Jones, MD
Assistant Professor of Neurology, Director, Child Neurology Residency Program, J401 Kentucky Clinic, Department of Neurology, University of Kentucky College of Medicine, Lexington, Kentucky 40536 United States. Email: Kimberly.Jones2@uky.edu

Victor Kieu, MD
PGY – 1 Pediatrics Resident, University of Kentucky College of Medicine, Kentucky Children's Hospital, Department of Pediatrics, 800 Rose Street, MN 472, Lexington, KY 40536 United States. Email: victor.kieu@uky.edu

Donita D. Lightner, MD
Assistant Professor of Neurology, J401 Kentucky Clinic, Department of Neurology, University of Kentucky College of Medicine, Lexington, Kentucky 40536 United States. Email: donita.lightner@uky.edu

Cori Morgan, APRN, FNP-C
Family Nurse Practitioner, L406 Kentucky Clinic, Department of Pediatrics, Kentucky Children's Hospital, University of Kentucky College of Medicine, Lexington, KY 40536 United States. E-mail: cearen2@uky.edu

Valeria I. Naranjo, MD
PGY – 3 Child Neurology Resident, J401 Kentucky Clinic, Department of Neurology, University of Kentucky College of Medicine, Lexington, Kentucky 40536 United States. E-mail: valeria.naranjo@uky.edu

Hatim Omar, MD, FAAP
Professor of Pediatrics and Obstetrics & Gynecology, Director of Adolescent Medicine and Young Parent programs, L412 Kentucky Clinic, Department of Pediatrics, Kentucky Children's Hospital, University of Kentucky College of Medicine, Lexington, KY 40536 United States. E-mail: haomar2@uky.edu

Jennifer Perry, LCSW
Social Worker Principal, L406 Kentucky Clinic, Department of Pediatrics, Kentucky Children's Hospital, University of Kentucky College of Medicine, Lexington, KY 40536 United States. E-mail: jenniferglass@uky.edu

Sharoon Qaiser, MBBS
Fellow Physician Child Neurology, J401 Kentucky Clinic, Department of Neurology, University of Kentucky College of Medicine, Lexington, Kentucky 40536 United States. E-mail: sharoon.qaiser@uky.edu

Mandakini Sadhir, MD
Associate Professor of Pediatrics, L411 Kentucky Clinic, Department of Pediatrics, Kentucky Children's Hospital, University of Kentucky College of Medicine, Lexington, KY 40536 United States. E-mail: m.sadhir@uky.edu

Kara Scott, APRN DNP CPNP-PC
L406 Kentucky Clinic, Department of Pediatrics, Kentucky Children's Hospital, University of Kentucky College of Medicine, Lexington, KY 40536 United States. E-mail: kara.scott@uky.edu

Taryn Solomon, RDN, LD, CNSC
L407 Kentucky Clinic, Department of Pediatrics, Kentucky Children's Hospital, University of Kentucky College of Medicine, Lexington, KY 40536 United States. E-mail: taryn.solomon@uky.edu

Stephanie Stockburger, MD
Associate Professor of Pediatrics, L407 Kentucky Clinic, Department of Pediatrics, Kentucky Children's Hospital, University of Kentucky College of Medicine, Lexington, KY 40536 United States. E-mail: stephanie.stockburger@uky.edu

Nikki Thaker, OMSIV
Edward Via College of Osteopathic Medicine, 2365 Kraft Drive, Blacksburg, VA 24060 United States. E-mail: nthaker@vt.vcom.edu

Chapter 17

About The Division of Adolescent Medicine, Kentucky Children's Hospital at The University of Kentucky, Lexington, Kentucky, United States of America

Kentucky Children's Hospital

The Kentucky Children's Hospital is the only facility in central and eastern Kentucky dedicated to the expert medical and surgical care of infants, children and adolescents. The University of Kentucky (UK) has a proud and distinguished history of providing comprehensive programs and innovative care to the children of the region. Although patients are referred from every county of the Commonwealth of Kentucky and from every adjacent state, the majority of patients are from the Bluegrass region around Lexington and from Appalachian counties in the eastern part of Kentucky. The Department of Pediatrics has provided service and education from the opening of UK College of Medicine in 1961.

The passion for teaching is palpable at the Kentucky Children's Hospital. Most years about 15% of our graduates or more choose to train in pediatrics. The University of Kentucky had one of the earliest combined Internal Medicine-Pediatrics residency program with "med-peds" graduates very well represented throughout the faculty. This, in addition to a strong adolescent medicine program, is among factors which have led to a focus upon adolescent and adult graduates of pediatric care from Kentucky Children's Hospital.

The approach at the Kentucky Children's Hospital (KCH) is focused on family-centered care. Full-time child life coverage, facilities for families to stay with children overnight, age-appropriate playrooms, children's library facilities, in-hospital school services, a dedicated television channel, a computer laboratory and many other features provide the special environment to provide the best of care for children. The Kentucky Children's Hospital includes a 12-bed Pediatric Intensive Care Unit, a 66 bed Level 3 Neonatal Intensive Care Unit, 44 acute care pediatric beds, a 26 bed normal newborn nursery, and an 8 bed short stay admissions/observation unit. KCH has grown from about 3,750 discharges per year in 2004 to about 5,400 in 2009.

Pediatric medical and surgical outpatient facilities are primarily located in the Kentucky Clinic, which is attached to the hospital. Each year, the pediatric clinic has over 46,000 patient visits. Of these, over 15,300 patient visits are in the general pediatric and continuity clinics, over 17,400 occur in the various subspecialty clinics. Kentucky Children's Twilight Clinic is open all but two days of the year in addition to the state-of –the-art pediatric emergency center.

Specialty care includes medical and surgical cardiac care, endocrinology, pediatric kidney disease, developmental pediatrics, pediatric allergy and immunology, solid organ transplantation, behavioral pediatrics, pediatric emergency medicine, intensive care pediatrics, neonatology, gastroenterology and hepatology, dysmorphology, biochemical genetics, pediatric rheumatology, oncology, hematology, infectious diseases, hospitalist care, adolescent medicine, adolescent gynecology, child neurology, pediatric surgery, pediatric orthopedics, pediatric imaging, child psychiatry, pediatric anesthesiology, pediatric otorhinolaryngology, speech disorders, pediatric pathology, pediatric physical medicine, pediatric neurosurgery and many other fields. The Young Parents Program is an innovative service of the Adolescent Medicine Division, which has been very successful. Many of these specialties cover outreach clinics throughout underserved Appalachian counties of Kentucky as well as in Lexington. New facilities are in preparation, because of the remarkable growth in clinical programs for children.

The growth of clinical programs and service capability has been matched by considerable growth in pediatric research at UK. Substantial programs in vascular biology and diabetes, pediatric inflammatory biology, molecular pediatrics, developmental biology, pediatric health policy research, epidemiology, prevention, cancer research and pediatric pharmacology are growing rapidly. The Kentucky Children's Hospital is located on the UK campus. Access to faculty in the other colleges including social sciences and humanities enhances the Kentucky Children's Hospital scholarly environment and provides unique opportunities for collaborative work.

As we approach our 50th year anniversary, we remain committed to improving the lives and health of young people of the Commonwealth and improving the future for their families.

Division of Adolescent Medicine

The Division of Adolescent Medicine was founded in 1998 to provide state of the art care for adolescent patients from all areas of the commonwealth of Kentucky, to serve as a state wide resource for education and training for local providers on adolescent issues, to study specific factors on the local level affecting youth in the state, to help teach medical students and residents and to provide community service to help improve teen future in the commonwealth.

The division provides comprehensive, holistic team approach to adolescents, where teens receive all aspects of care from mental health to routine care from a team of professionals including physicians, mental health providers, social workers, psychologists, nutritionists and nursing staff. One unique program within the division is the Young Parent Program, where pregnant teens are cared for throughout pregnancy then they and their babies are cared for together in the program.

The division is active in research with many peer reviewed articles published each year as well as several books and special journal editions.

In the community, the program has founded several grass route programs to help prevent youth suicide, teen pregnancy, accidental death and substance abuse among adolescents in Kentucky.

The division has provided more than 300 lectures, workshops, media events and teaching for community providers, parents, teachers and school counselors. It also provides advocacy work on behalf of teens with active work at the state legislative and executive government as well as local governments to help improve the lives of teens.

Collaborations

The Division of Adolescent Medicine collaborates locally with school boards, youth service centers, state and local governments, other universities and child advocacy centers as well as with regional adolescent medicine programs.

Internationally with the Institute for Child Health and Human Development in Israel, the Division of Adolescent Medicine at Santa Casa University, Brazil, Quality of Life Research Center and Nordic School of Holistic Health, Copenhagen, Denmark, Department of Applied Social Sciences, The Hong Kong Polytechnic University, Hong Kong.

The Vision

The vision of the Division of Adolescent Medicine is to improve the health and long term wellbeing of Kentucky Youth to grow into productive adults. We also invasion global work to help positive youth development worldwide.

Target Areas of Interests

The interest areas of the division are all aspects of youth development and adolescent health with focus on prevention and community involvement in collaboration on the local, national and global level with programs having the same goal.

Contact

Hatim Omar, MD, FAAP
Professor of Pediatrics and Obstetrics/Gynecology
Director of Adolescent Medicine & Young Parent programs
L412, Kentucky Clinic
Department of Pediatrics, Kentucky Children's Hospital
University of Kentucky College of Medicine
Lexington, KY 40536
E-mail: haomar2@uky.edu
Website: https://ukhealthcare.uky.edu/adolescent-medicine/

Chapter 18

About the Multiple Sclerosis program, Kentucky Neuroscience Institute (KNI) at the University of Kentucky, Lexington, Kentucky, United States

Kentucky Neuroscience Institute (KNI)

The Kentucky Neuroscience Institute (KNI) integrates the expertise of the University of Kentucky's neurology and neurosurgery clinicians and researchers. KNI is a referral center dedicated to providing comprehensive care to our patients with the most complex neurological conditions.

Neurosurgeons and neurologists at KNI diagnose and treat a wide spectrum of neurological conditions involving the brain, spine, nerves and muscles. Our team includes neurosurgeons, neurologists, neuropsychologists, therapists, nurses and other clinicians who use the most advanced surgical and medical treatments for brain, spinal cord, and nerve and muscle diseases and disorders. UK faculty also conduct cutting-edge clinical research and can offer innovative new treatment approaches. Our faculty are also training the next generation of health care providers and investigators. KNI is on the leading edge of patient care, research and education and puts the power of advanced medicine and an entire team of specialists to work on our patients' conditions.

Comprehensive Multiple Sclerosis Center

The University of Kentucky is a Comprehensive MS center provides care for patients living with MS. We provide a full range of services including diagnosis, treatment, and management of multiple sclerosis and related inflammatory conditions of the nervous system.

We are a physician lead team including but not limited to neurologists, psychiatrists, urologists, social work, nursing staff, physical therapy, and pharmacy. We have our own specialized pharmacy with two full time pharmacists who help provide medication support to our patients. MS is a complex disease affecting multiple domains, and provide a full range of supplementary services to address the patient's overall mood, energy level, functional capacity and wellness. We are actively involved in clinical trials, scholarly pursuits, and original research in an attempt to answer the unknown questions in MS. The University of Kentucky is the major teaching hospital for the commonwealth of Kentucky. The department of neurology is actively engaged in the teaching of medical students, and residents to equip the next generation of physicians. It is our goal to provide the highest level of care to those living with MS and their families in an attempt to alleviate suffering, and for our patients to live productive lives.

Contact

Joshua Chalkley, DO, MS
Assistant Professor of Neurology

J401 Kentucky Clinic
Department of Neurology
University of Kentucky College of Medicine
Lexington, Kentucky 40536
E-mail: Josh.Chalkley@uky.edu
Website: https://ukhealthcare.uky.edu/kni/

Chapter 19

About the National Institute of Child Health and Human Development in Israel

The National Institute of Child Health and Human Development (NICHD) in Israel was established in 1998 as a virtual institute under the auspices of the Medical Director, Ministry of Social Affairs and Social Services in order to function as the research arm for the Office of the Medical Director. In 1998 the National Council for Child Health and Pediatrics, Ministry of Health and in 1999 the Director General and Deputy Director General of the Ministry of Health endorsed the establishment of the NICHD.

Mission

The mission of a National Institute for Child Health and Human Development in Israel is to provide an academic focal point for the scholarly interdisciplinary study of child life, health, public health, welfare, disability, rehabilitation, intellectual disability and related aspects of human development. This mission includes research, teaching, clinical work, information and public service activities in the field of child health and human development.

Service and academic activities

Over the years many activities became focused in the south of Israel due to collaboration with various professionals at the Faculty of Health Sciences (FOHS) at the Ben Gurion University of the Negev (BGU). Since 2000 an affiliation with the Zusman Child Development Center at the Pediatric Division of Soroka University Medical Center has resulted in collaboration around the establishment of the Down Syndrome Clinic at that center. In 2002 a full course on “Disability” was established at the Recanati School for Allied Professions in the Community, FOHS, BGU and in 2005 collaboration was started with the Primary Care Unit of the faculty and disability became part of the master of public health course on “Children and society”. In the academic year 2005-2006 a one semester course on “Aging with disability” was started as part of the master of science program in gerontology in our collaboration with the Center for Multidisciplinary Research in Aging. In 2010 collaborations with the Division of Pediatrics, Hadassah Hebrew University Medical Center, Jerusalem, Israel around the National Down Syndrome Center and teaching students and residents about intellectual and developmental disabilities as part of their training at this campus.

Research activities

The affiliated staffs have over the years published work from projects and research activities in this national and international collaboration. In the year 2000 the International Journal of Adolescent Medicine and Health and in 2005 the International Journal on Disability and Human Development of De Gruyter Publishing House (Berlin and New York) were affiliated with the National Institute of Child Health and Human Development. From

2008 also the International Journal of Child Health and Human Development (Nova Science, New York), the International Journal of Child and Adolescent Health (Nova Science) and the Journal of Pain Management (Nova Science) affiliated and from 2009 the International Public Health Journal (Nova Science) and Journal of Alternative Medicine Research (Nova Science). All peer-reviewed international journals.

National collaborations

Nationally the NICHD works in collaboration with the Faculty of Health Sciences, Ben Gurion University of the Negev; Department of Physical Therapy, Sackler School of Medicine, Tel Aviv University; Autism Center, Assaf HaRofeh Medical Center; National Rett and PKU Centers at Chaim Sheba Medical Center, Tel HaShomer; Department of Physiotherapy, Haifa University; Department of Education, Bar Ilan University, Ramat Gan, Faculty of Social Sciences and Health Sciences; College of Judea and Samaria in Ariel and in 2011 affiliation with Center for Pediatric Chronic Diseases and National Center for Down Syndrome, Department of Pediatrics, Hadassah Hebrew University Medical Center, Mount Scopus Campus, Jerusalem.

International collaborations

Internationally with the Department of Disability and Human Development, College of Applied Health Sciences, University of Illinois at Chicago; Strong Center for Developmental Disabilities, Golisano Children's Hospital at Strong, University of Rochester School of Medicine and Dentistry, New York; Centre on Intellectual Disabilities, University of Albany, New York; Centre for Chronic Disease Prevention and Control, Health Canada, Ottawa; Chandler Medical Center and Children's Hospital, Kentucky Children's Hospital, Section of Adolescent Medicine, University of Kentucky, Lexington; Chronic Disease Prevention and Control Research

Center, Baylor College of Medicine, Houston, Texas; Division of Neuroscience, Department of Psychiatry, Columbia University, New York; Institute for the Study of Disadvantage and Disability, Atlanta; Center for Autism and Related Disorders, Department Psychiatry, Children's Hospital Boston, Boston; Department of Pediatric and Adolescent Medicine, Western Michigan University Homer Stryker MD School of Medicine, Kalamazoo, Michigan, United States; Department of Paediatrics, Child Health and Adolescent Medicine, Children's Hospital at Westmead, Westmead, Australia; International Centre for the Study of Occupational and Mental Health, Düsseldorf, Germany; Centre for Advanced Studies in Nursing, Department of General Practice and Primary Care, University of Aberdeen, Aberdeen, United Kingdom; Quality of Life Research Center, Copenhagen, Denmark; Nordic School of Public Health, Gottenburg, Sweden, Scandinavian Institute of Quality of Working Life, Oslo, Norway; The Department of Applied Social Sciences (APSS) of The Hong Kong Polytechnic University Hong Kong.

Targets

Our focus is on research, international collaborations, clinical work, teaching and policy in health, disability and human development and to establish the NICHD as a permanent institute in Israel in order to conduct model research and together with the four university schools of public health/medicine in Israel to establish a national master and doctoral program in disability and human development at the institute to secure the next generation of professionals working in this often non-prestigious/low-status field of work.

Contact

Joav Merrick, MD, MMedSci, DMSc
Professor of Pediatrics
Medical Director, Health Services, Division for Intellectual and Developmental Disabilities, Ministry of Social Affairs and Social Services, POB 1260, IL-91012 Jerusalem, Israel.
E-mail: jmerrick@zahav.net.il

Chapter 20

About the Book Series "Pediatrics, Child and Adolescent Health"

Pediatrics, child and adolescent health is a book series with publications from a multidisciplinary group of researchers, practitioners and clinicians for an international professional forum interested in the broad spectrum of pediatric medicine, child health, adolescent health and human development.

- Merrick J, ed. *Child and adolescent health yearbook 2011*. New York: Nova Science, 2012.
- Merrick J, ed. *Child and adolescent health yearbook 2012*. New York: Nova Science, 2012.
- Roach RR, Greydanus DE, Patel DR, Homnick DN, Merrick J, eds. *Tropical pediatrics: A public health concern of international proportions*. New York: Nova Science, 2012.
- Merrick J, ed. *Child health and human development yearbook 2011*. New York: Nova Science, 2012.
- Merrick J, ed. *Child health and human development yearbook 2012*. New York: Nova Science, 2012.

- Shek DTL, Sun RCF, Merrick J, eds. Developmental issues in Chinese adolescents. New York: Nova Science, 2012.
- Shek DTL, Sun RCF, Merrick J, eds. *Positive youth development: Theory, research and application.* New York: Nova Science, 2012.
- Zachor DA, Merrick J, eds. *Understanding autism spectrum disorder: Current research aspects.* New York: Nova Science, 2012.
- Ma HK, Shek DTL, Merrick J, eds. *Positive youth development: A new school curriculum to tackle adolescent developmental issues.* New York: Nova Science, 2012.
- Wood D, Reiss JG, Ferris ME, Edwards LR, Merrick J, eds. *Transition from pediatric to adult medical care*. New York: Nova Science, 2012.
- Isenberg Y. *Guidelines for the healthy integration of the ill child in the educational system: Experience from Israel.* New York: Nova Science, 2013.
- Shek DTL, Sun RCF, Merrick J, eds. *Chinese adolescent development: Economic disadvantages, parents and intrapersonal development.* New York: Nova Science, 2013.
- Shek DTL, Sun RCF, Merrick J, eds. *University and college students: Health and development issues for the leaders of tomorrow.* New York: Nova Science, 2013.
- Shek DTL, Sun RCF, Merrick J, eds. *Adolescence and behavior issues in a Chinese context.* New York: Nova Science, 2013.
- Sun J, Buys N, Merrick J. *Advances in preterm infant research.* New York: Nova Science, 2013.
- Tsitsika A, Janikian M, Greydanus DE, Omar HA, Merrick J, eds. *Internet addiction: A public health concern in adolescence.* New York: Nova Science, 2013.
- Shek, DTL, Lee TY, Merrick J, eds. *Promotion of holistic development of young people in Hong Kong.* New York: Nova Science, 2013.
- Shek DTL, Ma CMS, Lu Y, Merrick J, eds. *Human developmental research: Experience from research in Hong Kong.* New York: Nova Science, 2013.
- Rubin IL, Merrick J, eds. *Child health and human development: Social, economic and environmental factors.* New York: Nova Science, 2013.
- Merrick J, ed. *Chronic disease and disability in childhood.* New York: Nova Science, 2013.

- Rubin IL, Merrick J, eds. *Break the cycle of environmental health disparities: Maternal and child health aspects*. New York: Nova Science, 2013.
- Rubin IL, Merrick J, eds. *Environmental health disparities in children: Asthma, obesity and food.* New York: Nova Science, 2013.
- Rubin IL, Merrick J, eds. *Environmental health: Home, school and community.* New York: Nova Science, 2013.
- Merrick J, Kandel I, Omar HA, eds. *Children, violence and bullying: International perspectives.* New York: Nova Science, 2013.
- Omar HA, Bowling CH, Merrick J, eds. *Playing with fire: Children, adolescents and firesetting.* New York: Nova Science, 2013.
- Merrick J, Tenenbaum A, Omar HA, eds. *School, adolescence and health issues.* New York: Nova Science, 2014.
- Merrick J, Tenenbaum A, Omar HA, eds. *Adolescence and sexuality: International perspectives.* New York: Nova Science, 2014.
- Diamond G, Arbel E. Adoption: *The search for a new parenthood adoption*. New York: Nova Science, 2014.
- Taylor MF, Pooley JA, Merrick J, eds. *Adolescence: Places and spaces.* New York: Nova Science, 2014.
- Greydanus DE, Feinberg AN, Merrick J, eds. *Born into this world: Health issues.* New York: Nova Science, 2014.
- Greydanus DE, Feinberg AN, Merrick J, eds. *Caring for the newborn: A comprehensive guide for the clinician.* New York: Nova Science, 2014.
- Rubin IL, Merrick J, eds. *Environment and hope: Improving health, reducing AIDS and promoting food security in the world.* New York: Nova Science, 2014.
- Greydanus DE, Feinberg AN, Merrick J, eds. *Pediatric and adolescent dermatology: Some current issues.* New York: Nova Science, 2014.
- Roach RR, Greydanus DE, Patel DR, Merrick J, eds. *Tropical pediatrics: A public health concern of international proportions,* 2nd ed. New York: Nova Science, 2015.
- Merrick J, ed. *Child and adolescent health issues: A tribute to the pediatrician Donald E Greydanus*. New York: Nova Science, 2015.

- Feinberg AN. *A pediatric resident pocket guide: Making the most of morning reports*. New York: Nova Science, 2015.
- Greydanus DE, Patel DR, Pratt HD, Calles Jr JL, Nazeer A, Merrick J, eds. *Behavioral pediatrics*, 4th ed. New York: Nova Science, 2015.
- Merrick J, ed. *Disability, chronic disease and human development.* New York: Nova Science, 2015.
- Hegamin-Younger C, Merrick J, eds. *Caribbean adolescents: Some public health concerns.* New York: Nova Science, 2015.
- Merrick J, ed. *Adolescence and health: Some international perspectives*. New York: Nova Science, 2015.
- Omar HA. *Youth suicide prevention: Everybody's business.* New York: Nova Science, 2015.
- Greydanus DE, Raj VMS, Merrick J, eds. *Chronic disease and disability: The pediatric kidney.* New York: Nova Science, 2015.
- Merrick J, ed. *Children and childhood: Some international aspects.* New York: Nova Science, 2016.
- Shek DTL, Lee TY, Merrick J, eds. *Children and adolescents: Future challenges.* New York: Nova Science, 2016.
- Shek DTL, Wu FKU, Leung JTY, Merrick J, eds. *Adolescence: Positive youth development programs in Chinese communities.* New York: Nova Science, 2016.
- Merrick J, Greydanus DE, eds. *Sexuality: Some international aspects*. New York: Nova Science, 2016.
- Harel-Fisch Y, Abdeen Z, Navot M. *Growing up in the Middle East: The daily lives and well-being of Israeli and Palestinian youth.* New York: Nova Science, 2016.
- Greydanus DE, Malhotra D, Merrick J, eds. *Chronic disease and disability: The pediatric heart.* New York: Nova Science, 2016.
- Greydanus DE, Kamboj MK, Merrick J, eds. *Chronic disease and disability: The pediatric pancreas*. New York: Nova Science, 2016.
- Kamboj MK, Greydanus DE, Merrick J, eds. *Diabetes mellitus: Childhood and adolescence.* New York: Nova Science, 2016.
- Greydanus DE, Palusci VJ, Merrick J, eds. *Chronic disease and disability: Abuse and neglect in childhood and adolescence.* New York: Nova Science, 2016.
- Greydanus DE, Calles JL Jr, Patel DR, Nazeer A, Merrick J, eds. *Clinical aspects of psychopharmacology in childhood and adolescence*, 2nd ed. New York: Nova Science, 2016.

- Greydanus DE, Apple RW, White K, Merrick J, eds. *Children and youth: Post-traumatic stress disorder and motor vehicle crashes.* New York: Nova Science, 2017.
- Mazaba ML, Siziya S, Merrick J, eds. *Suicide: A global view on suicidal ideation among adolescents.* New York: Nova Science, 2017.
- Chow R, Merrick J, eds. *Adolescence: Bicycle and helmet use of adolescents and young adults.* New York: Nova Science, 2017.
- Shek DTL, Ma, CMS, Leung, JTY, Merrick J, eds. *Positive Youth Development. Long Term Effects in a Chinese Program.* New York: Nova Science, 2017.

Contact

Professor Joav Merrick, MD, MMedSci, DMSc
Medical Director, Medical Services
Division for Intellectual and Developmental Disabilities
Ministry of Social Affairs and Social Services
POBox 1260, IL-91012 Jerusalem, Israel
E-mail: jmerrick@zahav.net.il

SECTION THREE: INDEX

INDEX

M

N

O

P

Q

R

S

T

V

W